Weight-Resistance
YOGA

"Very impressive and necessary. I'm excited by this unique blend of Western-style strength training combined with the flexibility and meditative side of yoga. Popov's book is for all of us. It offers functional movement along with serentiy and mindfulness."

COLLEEN CRAIG, AUTHOR OF *PILATES ON THE BALL,*
ABS ON THE BALL, AND *STRENGTH TRAINING ON THE BALL*

"Melding hatha yoga and weight training into a blended practice, Max Popov shows us how these disciplines are not only completely compatible but also how each brilliantly supports the other's path of inquiry. By combining both, we go far beyond the individual benefits of stretching or strength and enter directly into the domain of a powerfully embodied spirituality."

WILL JOHNSON, AUTHOR OF *YOGA OF THE MAHAMUDRA*

"Bringing the yogic principle of mindfulness into all aspects of our lives is one of the ultimate goals of yoga. I recommend this book for anyone wishing to bring more spiritual depth to any physical exercise program."

BIFF MITHOEFER, AUTHOR OF *THE YIN YOGA KIT*
AND COAUTHOR OF *THE THERAPEUTIC YOGA KIT*

Weight-Resistance
YOGA

Practicing
Embodied Spirituality

Max Popov

Healing Arts Press
Rochester, Vermont • Toronto, Canada

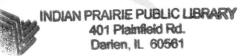

Healing Arts Press
One Park Street
Rochester, Vermont 05767
www.HealingArtsPress.com

Healing Arts Press is a division of Inner Traditions International

Note to the reader: *This book is intended as an informational guide. The remedies,
approaches, and techniques described herein are meant to supplement, and not to be a
substitute for, professional medical care or treatment. They should not be used to treat
a serious ailment without prior consultation with a qualified health care professional.*

Library of Congress Cataloging-in-Publication Data
Popov, Max.
 Weight-resistance yoga : practicing embodied spirituality / Max Popov.
   p. cm.
 Includes bibliographical references and index.
 ISBN 978-1-59477-390-7 (pbk.) — ISBN 978-1-59477-816-2 (e-book)
 1. Hatha yoga. 2. Weight training. I. Title.
 RA781.7.P66 2011
 613.7'046—dc23

2011032065

Printed and bound in the United States by P. A. Hutchison

10 9 8 7 6 5 4 3 2 1

Text design and layout by Virginia Scott Bowman
This book was typeset in Garamond Premier Pro and Gill Sans with Helvetica and
Gill Sans used as display typefaces

Illustrations in part 1 and chapter-opening illustrations in part 2 by Jacque Auger
Exercise illustrations in part 2 by Sarah Knotz
Illustrations on the title page, part-title spreads, and in part 3 by Henry Wojtas
Illustration on page 173 by Vince Serecin

To send correspondence to the author of this book, mail a first-class letter to the
author c/o Inner Traditions • Bear & Company, One Park Street, Rochester, VT
05767, and we will forward the communication, or contact the author directly at
MaxPopovWRY@aol.com or visit his website at **www.weight-resistanceyoga.com**.

for my slum goddess of the Lower East Side

CONTENTS

PART THREE

Meditations

MY JOURNEY
TO WEIGHT-RESISTANCE YOGA

In 1922, twenty-four-year-old Kolar Venkatesha Iyer founded the Hercules Gymnasium in Bangalore. It was the first commercial enterprise in India for bodybuilding, popularized in the West in the 1890s by Eugen Sandow, the German showman who originated flaunting one's muscular physique instead of showing off one's strength prowess. Iyer housed his gymnasium in what was once Tipu Sultan's summer palace—an ornate, two-storied, Indo-Islamic structure made of wood. Located in the rear of the state-owned building, the gymnasium consisted of two small rooms accessed by going around to the back and entering directly from the outside. At first there were only four students.

K. V. Iyer bestowed upon his students not only a muscular, harmonious physique—achieved through bell exercises and muscle control—but also the capacity to ward off chronic disease by virtue of the therapeutic practices of hatha yoga: *asana* (postures), *kriya* (cleansing techniques), *mudra* (seals), and *bandha* (locks). In so doing, he became the first person to combine what he called the "Cult of Body-building" and the "Hata-yoga Cult." "My aim in My System," he proclaimed

in 1930, "is to reconcile these two great systems to assure the future Culturist of robustness of health and beauty of limb and trunk."[1]

By the late 1930s, Iyer, who had become India's most famous bodybuilder and the owner of India's largest and most successful gymnasium, came to realize that the principal benefit of weight-resistance training isn't its ability to develop large muscles, with the attendant "pitfall of over-strain,"[2] but to make us "fit enough to accomplish each day's work with minimum fatigue and to remain active to a ripe old age."[3]

An Indian enthralled with the muscle-building systems of Europeans, yet proud of and indebted to the indigenous Indian practice of hatha yoga, Iyer had forged a dynamic system in which movements resisting opposing forces were coupled with movements surrendering to opposing forces—a combination that provided fitness and good health. About fifty years later, I unknowingly replicated his system when I began practicing and teaching a regimen that combined Western strengthening and yogic stretching exercises.

I first learned about Iyer in 1994 in David L. Chapman's biography of Sandow.

"The most important Indian physical culture instructor of the time," wrote Chapman, "[Iyer] attempted to blend Yoga, Hindu mysticism, and occidental physical culture into something uniquely his own."[4] This information electrified me. For the next dozen years, I researched Iyer's life and work. His mix of iconoclasm and asceticism influenced my weight-lifting practice. But before I even knew about Iyer, I'd already found my other lasting muse: the great yoga master Bellur Krishnamachar Sundararaja Iyengar, author of the groundbreaking encyclopedic manual of yoga poses *Light on Yoga*. Of his asana practice, the famous violinist Yehudi Menuhin said, "Yoga, as practiced by Mr. Iyengar, is a dedicated votive offering."[5]

Although I attended my first hatha yoga class in a bare loft located on Broadway in midtown Manhattan in the late 1960s, I only became immersed in hatha yoga in 1986 when I began taking classes with a dour, inspiring teacher at the first Iyengar Yoga Center of New York in Soho. Iyengar yoga demands unprecedented precision and élan, with careful attention paid to strict spinal alignment, using blocks, belts, and blankets to make accommodations. Marked equally by the finickiness and flamboyance of its founder, Iyengar yoga is a vigorous form of asana practice.

Several months after my immersion in Iyengar yoga, I took up strength training at a small, storefront gym, Natural Physique Centre, in the East Village. A skinny, withdrawn guy, I found myself among beefy men, with bald chests, and women, in skimpy spandex outfits, dedicated to pumping iron. What could be less like yoga than the glorification of aggressive muscular display (by mostly affable men and women) that I saw around me? Yet, what immediately struck me was that strength training—the stripped-down version of bodybuilding—and yogic flexibility training are inherently similar. Both exercise regimens seek to attain and maintain muscle and joint fitness. Both require a vast degree of resolve in order to expend great physical effort and overcome discomfort and fatigue.

In fact, I realized, the basic differences in fitness (the ability to perform muscle and joint work satisfactorily) between weight-resistance training (contracting muscles to increase strength) and yogic weight-surrender training (elongating muscles to increase flexibility) are complementary: together they make a whole and complete fitness regimen. They seem incompatible only because of the way weight-resistance training is commonly performed—something, I knew, that could be changed.

What I saw around me in the gym were weight-resistance exercises performed with sloppy form—movements that were careless, rushed, and spasmodic. To avoid this way of performing, I simply applied to my strengthening exercises the principles that I learned in yoga class: using moderately slow, controlled movements, maintaining postural alignment as much as possible, concentrating on moving a part of the body while expanding attention to the entire body, and breathing rhythmically. With the result that I established a weight-resistance routine—what I started thinking of as a weight-resistant yoga practice—that not only was efficient, safe, and effective but also, I discovered, facilitated mindfulness.

Mindfulness involves a directed (not just a vague) awareness of what we're doing. Knowing that left untended, the mind, like a neglected child, becomes unruly, yogins seek to empty the mind of all thoughts that are impediments to full concentration. We notice when our mind wanders to nagging or fleeting thoughts—such as regret over a flare-up of anger, or anxiety over meeting a deadline, or the desire for a painful exercise to be over. Then we bring our attention back to the minute demands of the task at hand and in so doing cultivate calmness and contentment.

These exercise principles taken from my yogic stretching practice, as well as the principles inherent in my strengthening practice, make up the exercise guidelines in part one of this book. They will enable you to perform the strengthening exercises, in part two, as mindful hatha yoga.

In the late 1980s, my weight-resistance yoga practice gradually turned meditative. The meditations weren't traditional. The subject wasn't fire or Vishnu or some other god (whom I imagined being in the lotus of the heart). Nor were the meditations New Age guided imagery. The subject wasn't a placid picture of me sitting in a flower garden or some such idyllic scene. The meditations were evoked by the movements of my body against resistance. I found myself comprehending realities behind everyday life through performing such exercises as bending backward on the Roman chair (sensing the poignancy of my mortality in my spinal bones); lifting a weight off my shoulders (bringing awareness to how all activities involve resisting and surrendering to the wearying pull of gravity); or toe raises (realizing that the restless quest for novelty can be replaced with the satisfactions of pleasurable repetition)—in other words, through becoming absorbed in my embodied being. I had no context for these experiences. Until I read B. K. S. Iyengar's *The Tree of Yoga,* published in 1988.

As commonly interpreted, hatha yoga, as explicated in Patanjali's *Yoga Sutras,* the foundational text of yoga, consists of a series of eight steps: *yama* (observing certain restraints), *niyama* (observing certain disciplines), *asana* (performing exercises), *pranayama* (breathing rhythmically), *pratyahara* (calming the senses), *dharana* (concentrating on aspects of bodily movement), *dhyana* (grasping the body—in its stillness, stability, and movement—as a whole) and *samadhi* (all concern with the self disregarded, comprehending the realities that are hidden during everyday life). In *Tree of Yoga,* however, Iyengar declared that all of the aspects of hatha yoga are intrinsically present in asana: "Within the one discipline of asana all the eight levels of yoga are involved, from yama and niyama through to samadhi."[6] An apprehension of the true nature of reality, Iyengar recognized, manifests itself in asana practice.

Yoga teacher and scholar Karl Baier elaborated on Iyengar's reflection on his asana practice as a kind of philosophizing. "Philosophy on *asana,*" Baier said, "tries to explain the experience of *asana.* . . . Philosophy on *asana* is . . . not mere abstract theory but is grounded in the philosophy within *asana,* which happens deep within the heart of the pose and enlightens the whole practice."[7] I began to keep a journal of my weight-resistance yoga experiences. This process helped me clarify my attempt at creating (what I now realized was) a philosophy on weight-resistance yoga exercises—a philosophy consisting not of a removed examination of reality but of meditations on reality manifested while performing the exercises.

It was Svatmarama's fifteenth-/sixteenth-century *Hatha Yoga Pradipika* (Light on Hatha Yoga), the first hatha yoga manual, that provided me with a model of a spun-out meditation—specifically, the exquisite and deeply perceptive long riff on *anahata nada* (sounds made without contact between two objects, located by Svatmarama within the body and handily accessed by blocking the ears) in chapter four. Infused with Tantra and alchemy, the *Hatha Yoga Pradipika* is certainly idiosyncratic: with its promotion of weird sexual practices, advocacy of barbaric hygienic procedures, claims of superhuman powers, tendency toward morbidity, and use of startling and vivid figures of speech, it's a screwy little book. And it's personal to Svatmarama: although a yoga manual, it reads (between the lines) like his diary or notebook.

Yet the *Hatha Yoga Pradipika* is eminently sensible and universal—and stirring. Whereas the *Yoga Sutras* is always prescriptive, the *Hatha Yoga Pradipika* is sometimes sublimely, beautifully descriptive. Svatmarama is so exquisitely attuned to bodily sensations that he describes the manifestation of happiness as "the *anahat* sounds, like various tinkling sounds of ornaments, being heard in the body."[8] Has there ever been a better description of what we may experience when we're perfectly happy—which means to say, when we transcend everyday reality?

In yoga, a practical philosophy, transcendence of the human condition is attained through the technique of meditation. I believe that this transcendence—what in yoga is called liberation—constitutes experience, and, therefore is not ineffable. (All experience can be described, no matter how inadequately.) The illuminations of meditation (apprehensions, say, of immediacy or the oceanic) can be and should be articulated. In fact, like Svatmarama, I believe that a critical part of a yoga teacher's role is to express these states of illumination.

Accordingly, meditative reflections—clarified and refined versions of my journal entrees—can be found in part three of this book. You can read a meditation outside the session (say, in the evening before sleep or in the morning upon waking) as a model for a self-reflective and contemplative approach to the weight-resistance training session, serving to stimulate your unique meditations. Or you can read brief passages at the beginning of the session in order to introduce a theme, which can be literally fleshed out through the practice. The theme will only have impact, though, if you sense it in your body through direct experience.

Whenever a comprehension of realities behind everyday life doesn't occur in a session, don't strain after it. After all, revelation is essentially unbidden. It comes by itself. But that doesn't mean that the effort put into weight-resistance yoga practice is futile. A deepened sense of reality can only be attained by practice. Becoming skilled at a weight-resistance yogic exercise, like learning an asana or memorizing a *shastra,* may take years; it involves working on the details of subtle and gross movements, over and over again. Perfecting the exercises, though, facilitates total withdrawal from (necessary) quotidian concerns by demanding full absorption. Emptying our mind of all ruminations through this total absorption in the exercises—making our mind still and receptive—allows for the possibility of opening up to transcendent Being.

ACKNOWLEDGMENTS

To my once and forever yoga teacher Judy Brick Freedman, who initiated me on my yoga journey; to the seer Will Johnson, who put in a good word for me at Inner Traditions; to my godsend, my Inner Traditions project editor, Laura Schlivek, who shepherded my book to publication; to my illustrators, Jacque Auger, Sarah Knotz, Henry Wojtas, and Vince Serecin, who created beautiful art—thank you all for putting up with me!

THE PATH OF WEIGHT-RESISTANCE YOGA

When I tell my fellow weight-surrender yogins (devotees of asana practice) that I also practice weight-resistance yoga, they usually say to me, "What's that?" When I explain that it's a yogic discipline for performing strengthening exercises instead of flexibility exercises, they may say, "I'm strong enough. I don't need to strength train." Or: "My yoga practice provides sufficient strength training. I don't need anything else." Or: "I recognize the need for separate strength training. But I'm so put off by weight lifting, I'd never do it." Or: "I already do some weight lifting. I don't need to do anything different." And if I'm able to gingerly convince them otherwise, they may still triumphantly say, smiling, "Yoga isn't merely exercise for achieving fitness, you know. It's a discipline for achieving liberation of self. How can your weight-resistance yoga match that?!" I'll try to fully address all these matters the best I can.

Why Weight-Surrender Yogins Need Strength Training

Our lives are filled with somewhat difficult physical actions. Just consider those commonly done at home: scrubbing a bathroom floor, picking up a child, rearranging furniture, opening a pickle jar, climbing stairs, taking down a clay hanging planter, stuffing a suitcase, opening a window, getting up from a couch, placing a box of clothes at the top of a closet.

All these actions involve movement against resistance. Muscles serve movement by producing or controlling the motion of a bony lever around a joint axis. For example, we pick up a basket of laundry from a table by bending our forearm (the bony lever) at the elbow joint (the joint axis), and we carefully place the basket down on a table by controlling, or slowing down, the straightening of the forearm.

Muscles also provide joint stability. A stable joint enables us to generate movement in the first place (a stable base is necessary for producing movement of a bony lever around a joint axis); to oppose external forces (occasionally, a strong wind, a crushing crowd, or the like, but most commonly, gravity); and to achieve optimal posture. For example, we avoid slouching by aligning the muscles of our neck, as well as our upper back, shoulders, and other muscles.

The strength training of weight-resistance yoga makes it easier for us to move (to push, pull, lift, and lower things; to stand up and sit down; and to walk and run) and to withstand being moved by outside forces. If the maximum weight that we can lift is fifteen pounds, then carrying a fifteen-pound basket of laundry takes maximum effort. If we increase our arm strength so that we can lift thirty pounds, carrying the same basket of laundry requires only half of our available muscle force, enabling us to perform the task with half the effort. If we've been sitting at a desk all day, our neck strength commonly decreases by about 30 percent by early evening due to the fatigue of holding our fifteen-pound head erect. If we increase the strength of our neck, as well as our upper back, shoulders, and other parts of our body, sitting up straight at the dining room table becomes less difficult.

Why the Strength Training of Weight-Surrender Yoga Is Insufficient

Many weight-surrender yogins believe there's no need to perform separate strengthening exercises because performing yoga postures, while focusing on increasing flexibility, also provides sufficient strengthening. But the strength conditioning provided by yoga flexibility exercises is inadequate.

During strength training, which employs measured resistance, the body responds to the demands of the force needed to overcome a greater-than-usual amount of resistance by making adaptations. In weight-resistance yoga, the amount of resistance is uniformly set at about 80 percent of one's maximum capacity—an intensity that stresses the muscles safely, efficiently, and effectively. In contrast, the strengthening aspect of asana practice is incidental and haphazard. It's a kind of casual calisthenics. For most of us, calisthenics—the manipulation of body weight to gain more strength—is an inadequate method of strengthening because our body isn't necessarily the optimal resistance for making strength gains: it may be too heavy (risks injury), too light (is inefficient), or unwieldy (is ineffective).

Asana practice is a particularly inadequate form of calisthenics. It doesn't use apparatus (such as a slant board, pull-up bar, or dip bar) to provide optimal direction and range of motion for using the body as weight resistance. It doesn't incorporate repetitions against the body as weight resistance. And it doesn't adequately stress dynamic, or moving, contractions (shortening of muscles by moving bony segments). Holding a freestanding yoga pose once by isometric, or static, contractions (shortening of muscles without moving bony segments)—which can be quite arduous—can provide some strengthening. But it's hardly effective for the strengthening necessary to carry out even the prosaic strength activities of daily life, especially as we get older.

How the Strengthening of Weight-Resistance Yoga Complements the Stretching of Weight-Surrender Yoga

Weight-resistance yoga develops a remarkable degree of flexibility, which is the capacity of a joint to move fluidly through its full range of motion. This is due to the practice's comprehensive use of the principle of reciprocal innervation: when the muscles primarily involved in causing a movement (called agonists) shorten, or contract, the muscles primarily involved in preventing the movement (called antagonists) elongate, or relax. By performing pairs of exercises for opposing (agonist and antagonist) muscle groups through a wide range of motion in a great variety of directions, weight-resistance yogins methodically increase not only strength but also flexibility. In fact, I sometimes treat my strength routine as a flexibility routine composed of exercises that begin with a brief static stretch of the agonist muscle group (in preparation for the first positive movement) and are followed by controlled dynamic stretches of the antagonist muscle group (during the positive movement phases of the repetitions). But this flexibility, no matter how thorough and balanced, doesn't by any means match that of weight-surrender yoga.

Weight-resistance yogins need the flexibility provided by weight-*surrender* yoga, just as much as weight-surrender yogins need the strength provided by weight-*resistance* yoga. Weight-resistance yoga and weight-surrender yoga complement each other.

How Weight-Resistance Yoga Is a Yogic Discipline for Fitness

Even when they recognize the need for strength training, many weight-surrender yogins can't bring themselves to perform strength-training exercises because they're put off by weight lifting. And with good reason. As anyone who has looked around in a gymnasium can testify, the weight-lifting milieu is largely made up of grunting men, red-faced and straining, using herky-jerky movements to propel heavy weights while performing multiple sets to bulk up the glamour muscles. Some weight-resistance yogins do actually perform strength-training exercises. But, having learned how to perform them from observing those around them in the gym, they feel that nothing about the way they strength train is compatible with their yoga practice. And they're right. But there's an entirely different way to perform weight-resistance exercises.

Process: Making Slow and Controlled Movements with Full Concentration

Weight-resistance yogins perform each exercise moderately slowly, with care and control—in other words, with full concentration. We perform approximately twelve to fifteen separate exercises, one time each per session. Over a week, we perform varied routines that systematically strengthen the muscles that produce all the major joint movements.

Purpose: Improving Everyday Life

Although its primary physiological adaptation is an increase in muscle strength, weight-resistance yoga doesn't dramatically increase muscle strength or, for that matter, size, local endurance (which applies to specific muscles), or power. It's designed to aid the healthy adult (i.e., one without disease or orthopedic limitations) seeking fitness—not the competitive (or even casual) bodybuilder and Olympic-style weight lifter or other elite athletes. Its benefits, achieved in collaboration with weight-surrender yoga, are decidedly unglamorous: performing common strength and flexibility activities nearly effortlessly, attaining comfortable postural alignment while sitting and standing, moving with ease, and preventing injury and illness.

Strength and Flexibility Activities of Daily Living

Often what enables us to perform a physical task is aggregate muscle action: muscles working in groups to perform an activity. Taking down a large ceramic serving bowl from the corner of the top cupboard shelf may involve twisting, reaching, grasping, and lowering movements that demand the coordination of muscles of the hand, wrist, arm, shoulder, back, and abdomen. Taking a bag of groceries from a car trunk involves bending, grasping, and lifting movements that engage not only the muscles of the arms but also of the calves, knees, upper legs, lower back, and abdomen. Both of these common activities entail a subtle interaction of strength and flexibility.

Although the type of joint movement is the same for all people, the force and range of movement differ considerably in different people. The vigor and extent of movement depend on the strength and flexibility of each person's ligaments and muscles. We can increase these capacities through regular weight-resistance and weight-surrender yoga practice, making daily strength and flexibility activities easier.

Postural Alignment

Resisting the constant pull of gravity toward the center of Earth, our bony skeleton supports our fleshy body. Muscles, tendons, ligaments, and fascia keep the bony segments aligned at their contacting surfaces, the joints. (Without muscles and connective tissue, the skeleton would collapse into a pile of bones.) Standard (i.e., ideal) posture is the state of skeletal balance that allows muscles to remain at their optimal resting alignment—neither shortened nor lengthened—and affords optimal positions for internal organs.

Looking at people around us while walking down the street, we see that standard posture is rare. Most people are bent over to some degree. If even slight deviations from standard posture aren't regularly corrected, they worsen over time, eventually causing a myriad of problems—not only of the musculoskeletal tissues (e.g., knotted up muscles, lower-back pain, fatigue, and proneness to injuries) but also of the organ systems (e.g., poor digestion, labored breathing, and increased susceptibility to respiratory ailments).

When bones are in alignment, muscles don't have to strain to help the bones hold up the body's weight, and organs of the trunk can function properly. The key to alignment is structural balance of the skeleton: equal pull of muscles located on opposite sides of a joint. Muscle imbalance is often due to overly lengthened (weak) muscles and overly shortened (tight) muscles. Weight-resistance yoga strengthens weak muscles, and weight-surrender yoga stretches tight muscles.

Mobility

Some of the challenging physical actions that pervade our lives make extra demands on our heart and lungs, whether briefly or over a long period of time. Some examples are running to catch a bus, climbing stairs, dancing, playing soccer, raking leaves, briskly walking, and bicycling. Therefore, a complete fitness program includes aerobic as well as strength and flexibility exercises. By stimulating the cardiorespiratory system more than everyday activities do, aerobic exercise provides the capacity to perform moderate-to-vigorous levels of common locomotive actions without undue fatigue.

Through providing strengthening exercises for the lower limbs, trunk, and upper limbs, weight-resistance yoga aids aerobic training, such as running and swimming, by increasing speed and endurance while reducing fatigue. These benefits, in turn, help maintain good form and avoid injury.

Performing the static stretches of weight-surrender yoga before an aerobic workout does not prevent overuse injuries and may even hinder performance; nevertheless, practicing weight-surrender yoga on a regular basis prevents injuries caused by persistently tight muscles (e.g., inelastic hamstring muscles).

Injury and Illness Prevention

We routinely apply force to put an object at rest into motion—to open a dresser drawer and take out socks, say, and then to shut the drawer. Daily activities like this are so unremarkable that we barely give them a thought until we're hampered or incapacitated by injury or illness. A breakdown of physical capacity can be alarming, even—or, perhaps, especially—when it affects the small tasks that we take for granted. It's an understandable cause for despair.

By increasing joint mobility, stability, range of motion, and balance, weight-resistance yoga helps prevent injuries (e.g., lower-back strain from lifting, strain to the middle and lower trapezius from habitually poor posture, overuse knee injury from jogging, and hip sprain from falling).

Weight-resistance training keeps us not only injury free but also healthy. According to the American College of Sports Medicine (as presented in its position stand for resistance training for healthy adults), "Resistance training, when incorporated into a comprehensive fitness program, improves cardiovascular function, reduces the risk factors associated with coronary heart disease and non-insulin-dependent diabetes, prevents osteoporosis, may reduce the risk of colon cancer, promotes weight loss and maintenance, improves dynamic stability and preserves functional capacity and fosters psychological well-being."[1] To reduce the risk of injury and the incidence of several chronic diseases, a comprehensive exercise program also incorporates flexibility exercises along with aerobic endurance activities.

How Weight-Resistance Yoga Is an Ascetic Yogic Discipline

Daily life is more pleasurable when we can easily push and pull and lift and lower things; freely bend, extend, and twist; adroitly resist outside forces such as jostling crowds and the wind; stand and sit without effort; walk and run without difficulty; and be free of injury and chronic disease. As we get older, we come to appreciate being able to perform banal tasks without strain, an accomplishment usually taken for granted. We take delight in ordinary activities. And in so doing, we come to be thankful for all that we can do. Reason enough to practice weight-resistance yoga.

Purpose: Withdrawing from Everyday Life

But there is another, perhaps even more compelling reason for practicing weight-resistance yoga—one that centers on the experience of the session itself. Weight-resistance yoga always retains its prosaic function as a strength-training program that uses a mix of dumbbells, barbells, machines, and the body to overcome resistance in order to improve everyday life. (This first stage of the practice begins immediately and takes about six months to attain mastery. Some students are satisfied with just this stage.)

But weight-resistance yoga, like weight-surrender yoga, is primarily a discipline for achieving liberation of self. More than a period of time set aside for fitness goals, the weight-resistance yoga session is also a welcome refuge from our stressful daily lives in which we must, for example, rush to get our kids to school or work overtime to get a report done.

The weight-resistance yoga session is a haven because it brings to strengthening exercises the same attentiveness and care that weight-surrender yoga brings to stretching postures. Discrete movements against resistance are performed within a context of stability and stillness and are coordinated with rhythmic breathing.

By placing emphasis on focused absorption in the body's complex movements during strengthening exercises, the weight-resistance yoga session lends itself to emptying the mind of everyday preoccupations. From this mindfulness, without our even trying, tranquillity emanates. (This second stage of the practice begins at about the third month.) Some students are perfectly satisfied with reaching only this stage. For many, I suspect, this will be the first time they actually look forward to practicing strength training rather than having it over with!

Purpose: Transcending Everyday Life

But the weight-resistance yoga session is more than an untroubled time away from the stress of everyday life. It's a time for meditating on the embodied experience of calmly performing strengthening exercises. (This third stage begins at about the ninth month. Attaining it requires first mastering the previous two stages.). As such, the session becomes a period devoted to the transformation of everyday life. Ordinarily, we must constantly attend to commonplace realities, such as time regulated by watches and calendars, schedules and deadlines. In this contemplative state, weight-resistance yogins comprehend realities ordinarily hidden during everyday life, such as time without beginning or end.

In one of the three foundational texts of hatha yoga, *Gheranda-Samhita* (Gheranda's Collection), from the late seventeenth or possibly early eighteenth century, Gheranda advised his disciple Chanda Kapali not to practice yoga "in the midst of a crowd" (unless it were like minded). "The curious will trouble you," he cautioned. "And distract you," he might have added. Gheranda recommended that "one erect a small hut, and around it let one raise walls" for practicing yoga.[2] Alas, for various reasons, most of us can't construct a small building with strength-training equipment on our property (or even install something like it in our basement) for practicing weight-resistance yoga. We have to go to the local gymnasium. There we have access to equipment, but—the unwelcome tradeoff—we are sometimes assaulted by loud bodybuilders and a blaring radio or television.

Someday there will be elegant and placid yoga centers for practicing weight-resistance yoga (along with weight-surrender yoga)—settings that facilitate, rather than militate against, our focusing on the complex movements against resistance, emptying our mind of everyday realities, and filling our soul with comprehensions of deeper realities. But until that time, we must bear in mind (more than usual!) that during weight-resistance yoga practice, our body itself is a dwelling—a spiritual dwelling, at that. The sage Gorakhnath chastened us to meet exactly this challenge: "How can the yogis who do not know their body as a house presided over by divinities attain perfection in yoga?"[3]

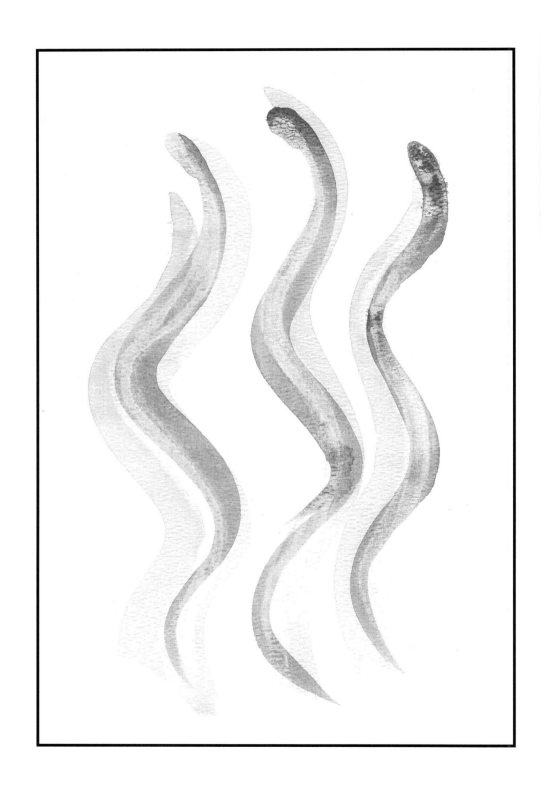

PART ONE

· · · · · · · · ·

Exercise Guidelines

For all of us who strength train, the physiological process is the same: our body responds to the demands of the force needed to overcome a greater than usual amount of resistance by making adaptations. We get stronger. But types of strength training vary. Weight-resistance yoga is a form of high-intensity training, the protocol developed by Arthur Jones, the founder of Nautilus, in the 1970s. The fundamental strength principles of weight resistance yoga include a high level of effort, 8–12 repetitions, a moderately slow lifting cadence, a relatively brief session consisting of single sets of approximately twelve exercises, and a schedule that allows a day between sessions for the parts of the body that have been worked. The basic goal of weight-resistance yoga is to provide adequate strength for everyday activities.

What primarily distinguishes weight-resistance yoga from other strength-training programs (even other high-intensity training workouts), though, is its emphasis on quietly performing relatively simple (yet exacting) movements against resistance made within stillness and stability and coordinated with rhythmic breathing. I think of these practices—when carried out with full concentration—as refusals to give in to our habitual inclinations: refusals to be slapdash, distracted, self-absorbed, unrhythmic, and fragmented. In our unwillingness to subject our body to exertion other than through tranquilly dwelling within our body, we make our practice a means of transcending everyday life, of opening ourselves up to Being.

1

IMMERSION

The weight-resistance yoga session is a period of quiet contemplation set apart from our hurried, anxious, noisy lives. During this time we shed our habitual patterns of behavior to tranquilly immerse ourselves in transformational rituals: *anjali mudra,* breathing exercises, strengthening exercises, and *Savasana.*

Taking Off Your Shoes

Optimally, we should practice weight-resistance yoga in a well-equipped, elegant, and tranquil room that is part of a hatha yoga center designed as a dwelling for transcending everyday existence. However, we consider wherever we practice weight-resistance yoga as a sacred space, a retreat from the everyday world. Accordingly, we treat the space with reverence.

Instruction
Before entering the weight-resistance yoga room of a hatha yoga center, remove your shoes and socks, and leave them by the entrance. Quietly walk in.

Anjali Mudra

Before initiating the exercises, we perform anjali mudra. Although considered a sacred hand gesture, anjali mudra is actually a whole-body position.

Instruction
To perform anjali mudra while standing, plant your feet squarely on the floor, parallel and slightly apart. Lift your kneecaps, and stretch the back of your knees. Keep your thighs fairly tight. Lift your spine, without flattening the natural curves of your back. Spread your shoulders to open your chest. Bring your shoulders down. Lift your head, thereby releasing tension in your neck.

Placing your hands together at the center of your chest, tenderly press your thumbs into your breastplate, or sternum, the flat bone that contributes to providing the armature that protects two vital organs—the heart and lungs—by connecting the seven true ribs and serving as an attachment site for the chest muscles. Draw your palms firmly together, extend your fingers until they're pointing upward, and lift your elbows until your forearms align with your wrists.

Gently and briefly bow your head without moving your shoulders or back (fig. 1.1).

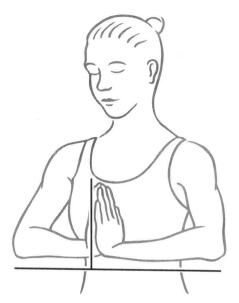

Fig. 1.1. Anjali mudra

In performing anjali mudra, this timeless position of composure, we establish calm and clarity for the time of our ensuing exercise practice.

Pranayama

In our everyday life, we routinely breathe without willed effort. During the weight-resistance yoga session, however, we meddle in our breathing by practicing pranayama, regulation of the breath.

Instruction

For this preparatory pranayama, inhale deeply and noisily through your nostrils with something like a hissing sound, hold your breath by constricting your throat, and then audibly, slowly, and fully exhale through your nostrils. Repeat a total of three times.

This attentiveness to the breath—a discernment of the subtle aspects of breathing—is further preparation for the turning inward that takes place during our practice.

Performing a Series of Strengthening Exercises

The primary activity of the weight-resistance yoga session is performing strength-training exercises. To ensure that our exercise routines are efficient, effective, and safe, we use various equipment (dumbbells, machines, benches, and such); perform single sets of a relatively small number of repetitions; execute a great variety of strength-conditioning exercises at an intensity that demands mighty exertion against gravitational and mechanical resistance.

Repetition: The repetition is one complete movement of a strength-training exercise. The repetition is composed of two phases: a concentric muscle contraction (which initiates the movement) and an eccentric muscle contraction (which controls the release of the movement). For example, during shoulder joint adduction (downward movement of the upper arm from the side), pulling a bar down from overhead to the sternum and returning the bar from the sternum to overhead is one repetition.

Instruction

Perform 8–12 repetitions per exercise.

Set: The set is a number of repetitions performed without interruption during a strength-training exercise. For example, during shoulder joint abduction (upward movement of the upper arm out to the side), lifting dumbbells from near the shoulders to overhead and lowering the dumbbells back to the shoulders, ten times continuously, is one set of ten repetitions.

Instruction

Perform each set only once.

Exercise Routine: The exercise routine is a previously established variety of strength-training exercises performed with short interruptions. The exercise routine typically consists of about twelve to fifteen exercises that take less than an hour to perform. For example, four exercises for the shoulder joint, two exercises for the elbow joint, and four exercises for the shoulder girdle is one upper-body exercise routine.

Instruction

Perform an exercise routine that consists of a great variety of exercises.

The exercises are performed in an alert and purposeful trance. Carried out in this way, they become a primary vehicle for opening ourselves up to Being.

Housekeeping

Wherever we reside, even in a prison or convent cell, our living space demands a certain amount of housekeeping.

Instruction

In this place where you've temporarily taken up residence to perform weight-resistance yoga, use the equipment with care. Clean the machines after using them. Routinely put back dumbbells, barbells, weight plates, and other equipment where they're stored.

We do all this in part as members of a community, to fulfill our obligations to others, and in part as spiritual beings, to preserve the sacred nature of the space.

Savasana

The session ends with Savasana, or Corpse Pose.

Instruction

Move to a room for resting or meditative postures, another sacred space in the hatha yoga center. Here place your body in Savasana. Lie on your back. Your feet should be about a foot and a half apart and falling away from each other. Place your hands by your sides. Close your eyes. Systematically move your attention through your body, from feet to head, alternately contracting and releasing parts of the body. Let your body soften and lengthen. Surrender to what you've been mightily resisting during the entire exercise routine: the pull of gravity (or some mechanical substitute) on your body. Sense your body being drawn toward the center of Earth. Be content with all that has transpired during the session and during your life.

Through partaking of these specified, ordered, and ceremonial actions that make up the weight-resistance yoga session, we transcend everyday life.

2

SAFE AND EFFICIENT EFFORT

Dealing with Equipment

Dumbbells and barbells, benches and chairs, calisthenics apparatus, and machines are the yoga props of weight-resistance yoga. Used to adjust angles and levels of intensity, this equipment—like the blocks, straps, and blankets of weight-surrender yoga—enhances the effectiveness of exercises. But dealing with this equipment—before, during, and after performing an exercise—risks injury. So precautions must be taken.

Moving Free Weights and Weight Plates

Handling free weights and weight plates carelessly before and after performing an exercise may cause strains or sprains.

Instruction

Whenever you pick up, hold, carry, or put down a dumbbell, barbell, or weight plate, there is stress on the neck, shoulders, arms, and lower back. Some of the most common strength-training injuries are caused by such actions as bending over to place a dumbbell back on a rack while standing too far away or lifting a weight plate from a machine without bending the knees. Handle free weights and weight plates with deliberation and care.

Getting On and Off Benches and Calisthenics Apparatus

Getting on and off benches and entering and exiting calisthenics apparatus should be done with care. Even non-weight-bearing movements, such as climbing onto a decline abdominal bench or hopping down from a chin-up bar, may cause injury.

Adjusting Benches and Machines

Performing an adjustable bench exercise efficiently and safely involves setting up the appropriate angle, such as raising or lowering the back of a bench to a slight incline for the shoulder press.

Performing a machine exercise efficiently and safely sometimes involves adjusting multiple machine parts to properly position your body. Because each exercise involves the entire body, we must adjust the machine parts for the entire body. For example, for the chest press, parts must be adjusted not only for moving the arms but for keeping the trunk stabilized and the head and lower limbs still. For the knee extension, parts must be adjusted not only for moving the lower legs but also for keeping the upper legs and trunk stabilized and the head and upper limbs still. (Because some machines, no matter how well we adjust them, just won't exactly fit our body type or size, sometimes we must accommodate ourselves the best we can.)

Instruction

Alter the seat, knee pads, arm pads, sled, cable arms, and other adjustable parts of plate-loaded, cable-and-pulley, and lever-arm-and-cam machines for optimal use and safety. For example, when using a chest press machine, adjust the seat and back so you can sit with your back aligned, your knees squared, and your feet firmly on the floor (fig. 2.1). When using a knee extension machine, in order to inhibit

lurching with your lower back to initiate the movement, set the back so that you can sit with your trunk at a right angle to your upper legs and with your knees snuggly draped over the front of the seat (fig 2.2).

Using Safety Features

Most barbell benches and plate-loaded machines have safety features.

Instruction

Before using barbell benches and plate-loaded machines for the first time, practice using their safety features—such as

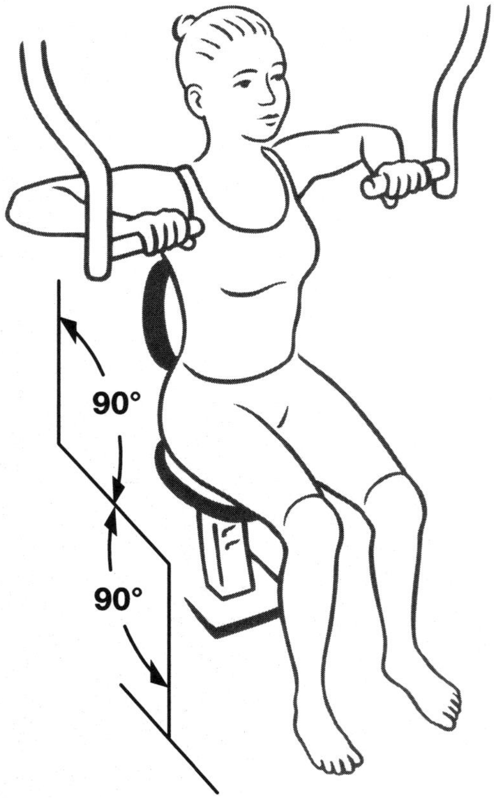

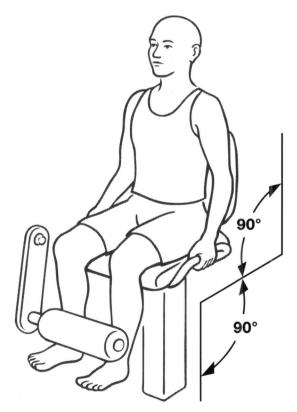

Fig. 2.1. Properly adjusted
chest press machine

Fig. 2.2. Properly adjusted
knee extension machine

the safety catch (the release/return mechanism) on the leg press machine and racks on the level bench press bench—so you can immediately return a weight when targeted muscles are exhausted.

Gripping Handles and Bars

The power of the clenched hand to grip a bar or handle or a dumbbell or barbell in performing a strength-training exercise (or to make a fist) is lessened when the wrist is in a flexed position (bent forward, say to 20 degrees) or even (to a lesser extent) in the neutral position (held straight). Optimal grip function occurs when the wrist is extended at an angle of fifteen to twenty degrees—a slightly upward position (fig. 2.3). Without this optimal tension, we can't completely tighten our fingers around the part that we hold, inhibiting our ability to fully push or pull.

Hyperextending the wrist (bending the wrist back beyond twenty degrees, say to 60 degrees) when gripping a bar, handle, or bell in performing a strength-training exercise may lead to developing lateral epicondylitis (tennis elbow), which causes pain with activities that require gripping (e.g., shaking hands, turning doorknobs, using hand tools, writing) or a combination of gripping and lifting (e.g., picking up groceries).

The overall goals of strength training are enhanced to some extent, however, by slightly *weakening* the hold on a bar by using the palm grip. The palm grip entails placing the thumb on the same side of a bar as the fingers. Its benefit is reducing the involvement of forearm muscles. Ordinarily, we want to recruit as many muscles as possible to pro-

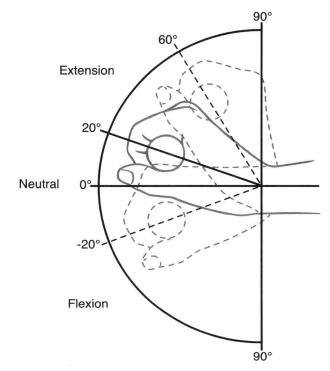

Fig. 2.3. Optimal grip angle

duce force. (By increasing the involvement of the forearm muscles, the standard grip, which entails placing the thumb on the opposite side of the fingers, is more effective for swinging a tool, such as a hammer.) But in strength training, we seek to isolate the muscles most involved in opposing resistance as much as possible. For example, using the palm grip for the bench press isolates the pectoral and triceps muscles—the targeted muscles.

Instruction

Use the palm grip when possible in order to isolate the muscles most involved in an exercise. Because the palm grip makes a barbell exercise somewhat unstable, slightly decrease the weight.

Assuming the Starting Position

An exercise shouldn't be initiated from the resting length of the part of the body that's the focus of the movement. When muscles move any one of the bony segments of the skeleton at their resting length, the muscles are exerting their greatest force at their most disadvantageous leverage, risking injury. For optimum leverage, the bony segment or segments about to be moved should always be set at a starting position slightly away from the resting position.

Instruction

Before initiating an exercise proper, position the about-to-be-moved bony segment or segments for optimal leverage—an inch or so away from the resting position— by making a short, quick movement, using a touch of momentum, if necessary. Examples of moving into this getting set position are slightly raising the forearms before beginning the standing biceps curl (fig. 2.4) and slightly raising the lower legs before beginning the knee curl (fig. 2.5).

Controlling Movement

Weight lifters commonly use poor form throughout or at the end of a set to resist a weight load that exceeds their strength capabilities. Routinely relying on poor form is inefficient and risks injury.

Throughout a Set

Some weight lifters use poor form throughout a set. Flinging dumbbells during the deltoid raise or snapping the handle back during

the low row uses excessive momentum— movement that can't be stopped at any point along the range of motion. By decreasing the time that a muscle is under tension, excessive momentum—like too much speed—limits

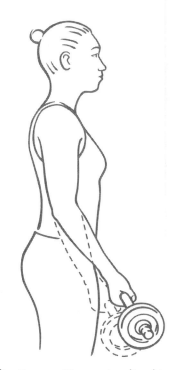

Fig. 2.4. Starting position—standing biceps curl

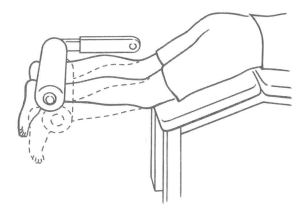

Fig. 2.5. Starting position—knee curl

muscle force, lessening an exercise's effectiveness. Unlike high speed, excessive momentum also stresses muscles and connective tissues at joint structures, which increases the risk of injury. For example, during the bench press, when the bar is raised with rapid thrusting, sometimes aided by bouncing the bar off the chest, and allowed to rapidly lower without restraint, we overstress the pectoralis major tendon where it attaches to the upper arm, causing inflammation.

Instruction

Unless you're doing power exercises (such as the snatch), which are correctly performed in an explosive manner, use a measured movement—relatively slow, deliberate, and careful—to oppose resistance throughout an exercise.

At the End of a Set

Other weight lifters use proper technique for most of a set but break correct form to accomplish the last two or three repetitions, when resisting the weight load becomes increasingly difficult.

Instruction

Lifting an excessively heavy weight load by breaking strict form, which relies on muscles that should be used for stabilizing the body, invariably leads to injury. When you're no longer lifting with correct form, stop.

To avoid having your form deteriorate, use a weight load that doesn't exceed your strength capabilities—one that allows you to apply consistent muscle force throughout the full range of motion without resorting to cheating movements (movements that deviate from traditional form, such as swinging weights or moving parts of the body to overcome a "sticking point," the weakest point in a range of motion). Although less weight will be resisted, the prime mover muscles will apply most of the force, providing more stimuli for them and lowering their risk for injury.

Although cheating is effective for competitive bodybuilders who are cautious (they don't exaggerate the deviation from correct form) and discriminating (they cheat selectively), adhere to strict form unless fatigue has placed you in danger of dropping a weight and you must put the weight down—right away—by any means.

It isn't difficult to spot good form: it's concise, formal, restrained, and graceful.

Manifesting Grace

When the demands of an exercise are difficult, weight lifters commonly adapt their body to enlist the assistance of nontargeted muscles or to maximize their mechanical leverage, and in so doing they make their movements awkward, contorted, and unsafe. For example, they lean into the exertion of a triceps pushdown exercise with a hunched-over posture. These bodily adaptations are often accompanied by strained facial expressions, even grimaces. These visual cues—body and facial language—when performing exercises reveal a state of agitation.

In the mid-twentieth century, the Indian

bodybuilder K. V. Iyer instructed his students:

> While you are using your limbs for exercises let them be used as gracefully as possible. There should be nothing ugly or contortioned either in your movements or in the facial expression. . . . When you flex your biceps let that be powerfully, yet, gracefully done. When you bend to a side or squat down or straighten yourself up, when you turn your head, or face, or knee, or feet, let each movement be done with all possible grace and power. Grace should become your second nature.[1]

Making our exertion smooth and fluid (forbidding it to be erratic and jerky), on the one hand, and skillful and regulated (instead of applying maximum force using momentum), on the other hand, not only makes an exercise efficient and safe but also facilitates calmness, the prerequisite for self-reflection and contemplation.

3

STILLNESS

Stilling our body during exercises allows us to turn our attention to the discrete strengthening movements of weight-resistance yoga. Indeed, the subtle, precise movements that produce force to oppose resistance can be flawlessly performed only within an absolute stillness of the body. One form of that stillness is relaxation, the absence of muscular tension or fidgetiness. (The other form is stabilization, discussed below.) Whether performing exercises while standing, sitting, lying down, or in some variation of these positions, weight-resistance yogins relax the parts of our body not involved in the targeted muscle action.

After taking a series of fussy preparatory actions (adjusting a machine, gripping handles or a bar, and taking a ready position), we relax these uninvolved parts in preparation for the movement against resistance. At this point, relaxation is a kind of poised stillness. It anticipates the movement. However, we keep these parts relaxed throughout the exercise, because muscular tension wastes energy, predisposing us to muscular tightness and fatigue, and extraneous movement interferes with focusing on the movement against resistance.

Difficult to achieve at first, stillness of inessential parts is attained by simultaneously loosening effort and controlling the natural tendency toward restlessness. Effortlessness and control cannot be acquired without adopting correct alignment of the skeletal bones, which allows for relaxation of the muscles. Poor posture strains muscles, which must exert constant tension to counteract the force of gravity pulling down misaligned skeletal bones. When we adjust our bony segments so they're stacked on each other in conformity to the pull of gravity, the supporting muscles— no longer required to produce effort—can relax. They can surrender to the pull of gravity. And they're less likely to absent-mindedly move about.

The key to lower-body alignment while standing is the pelvis. Two bony landmarks are used to assess pelvic alignment: the upper front of the bony rims around the waist (the anterior superior iliac spines, commonly mistaken as the location of the hip joints) and the midline joint of the pubic bones (the pubic symphysis). The pelvis is in a neutral position when the upper front of the rims are in the same horizontal plane as each

Anterior Superior Iliac Spines

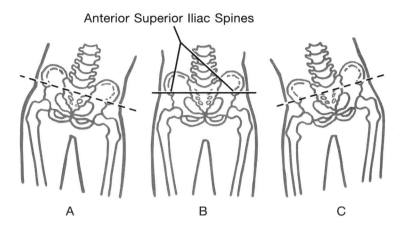

Fig. 3.1. Aligned pelvis in horizontal plane

other (fig. 3.1 B) and in the same vertical plane as the midline joint of the pubic bones (fig. 3.2 B).

The shoulder blades—not the back, chest or abdomen—may be considered the key to upper-body alignment. The upper body is in a neutral position when the upper vertebral border of the shoulder blades is parallel to the spine, positioned approximately three inches from the spine, flush against the thorax, and, where it meets the spine of the scapula, level with the third thoracic vertebra (fig. 3.3). Nevertheless, two tips for retaining ideal upper-body alignment are maintaining the natural curves of the back, and keeping constant the distance between the base of the

Anterior Superior Iliac Spine

Pubic Symphysis

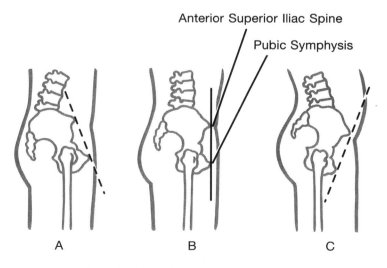

Fig. 3.2. Aligned pelvis in vertical plane

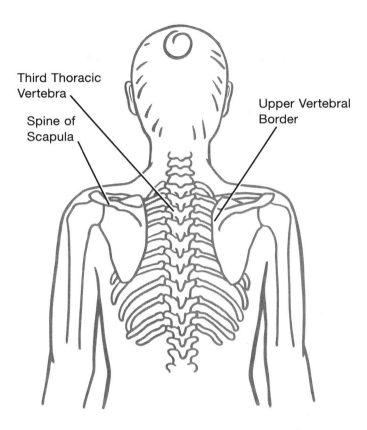

Third Thoracic
Vertebra

Spine of
Scapula

Upper Vertebral
Border

Fig. 3.3. Aligned shoulder blades

sternum (breast plate) and the midline joint of the pubic bones (the pubic symphysis).

In B. K. S. Iyengar's conceptualization of weight-surrender yoga, *Tadasana,* Mountain Pose, not *Padmasana,* Lotus Pose, is the embodiment of steadiness and ease. For this reason, Tadasana is more than the basic standing pose in Iyengar's system: it's the primary posture from which all other yoga postures are defined. Each asana is a variation of Tadasana. No matter what variations are demanded by the unique configurations of a pose, Tadasana, the expression of perfect alignment, is maintained as much as possible.

In weight-resistance yoga, just as in sports and medicine, all movement is defined as a variation of what is called the anatomical position, in which one stands erect, facing forward, the arms at the sides, the palms of the hands facing forward, and the feet parallel and close—a position that closely resembles Tadasana. Because the anatomical position also exemplifies perfect alignment, the anatomical position is maintained as much as possible no matter what variations are demanded by a strengthening exercise.

In fact, any configuration of the body during a weight-resistance yoga exercise is perceived as a temporary reconfiguration of the anatomical position. No matter how small the trace of it that remains in any given exercise, this upright position is the ground of immobility from which discrete movements arise. All movement is perceived as a temporary deviation from this immobility.

Weight lifters commonly strike a casual posture when performing exercises—slumped shoulders, forward head, and arched back during standing exercises; tilted tail bone supporting the torso during sitting exercises; and arched back and splayed knees while performing lying down exercises.

Weight-resistance yogins, in contrast, maintain standard alignment as much as possible in each exercise—keeping the spine erect, raising the sternum, expanding the chest, keeping the shoulders down and looking straight ahead. Carrying ourselves well throughout the exercise routine is an integral part of our workout.

Instruction

To ensure standard (that is, ideal) standing, sitting, and lying postures during the performance of weight-resistance yoga exercises, make any necessary skeletal adjustments.

When performing standing exercises, plant your feet firmly on the floor, centering your ankles, straightening (but not locking) your knees, and settling into a stable position with your pelvis aligned.

Sitting exercises demand greater vigilance than standing exercises, because sitting subjects the lumbar spine to a substantial compressive load. When performing sitting exercises, don't place your body weight on the tailbone (coccyx); instead, sit back on your haunches (ischial tuberosities).

During all exercises, lift your sternum (without arching your back), expand your chest, and gently pull your shoulder blades back and down, relaxing your shoulders. Pull the top posterior part of your head upward, release your neck, and lengthen your spine. Look straight ahead.

When the body is stilled in this way, we feel as if we can stand or sit or lie motionless for ages—as if, like a living ancient statue, we have been still for ages, calmly observing life's vicissitudes. In weight-resistance yoga, remaining immobile in this way allows the mind to fully and calmly concentrate on the strenuous movements to oppose resistance—the prerequisite for breaking down ordinary perceptions of self and the world.

4

MOVEMENT IN STILLNESS

Exerting Force

While keeping the parts of the body not involved in an exercise aligned and still and the face impassive, we perform weight-resistance yoga exercises by exerting force. There are three ways of exerting force: by concentric, eccentric, and isometric muscle contraction.

Concentric Muscle Contraction

During concentric, or positive, contraction, muscles are strengthened by overcoming resistance. Movement is involved: muscles attached to two bony parts are shortened, pulling one of the bony parts closer to the other. This production of force is ordinary, straightforward, and apparent.

Eccentric Muscle Contraction

But "the real peculiarity of muscle work," observes Steven Vogel, a historian of muscle, "turns on the relative strength and efficiency of negative work."[1] During eccentric, or negative, contraction, muscles are strengthened by giving in to resistance—begrudgingly. We hinder the rapid return of muscles to their resting length. Once again, movement

is involved: shortened muscles attached to the bony segments are lengthened slowly and with control, moving one of the body segments away from the other.

In weight-resistance yoga, eccentric contraction plays as critical a role as concentric contraction. Taking full advantage of eccentric contraction during strength training conditions us for everyday movement, of which eccentric contraction is an important component—for example, decelerating when abruptly stopping running, lowering a pot of soup to the table, and keeping the trunk of the body from swaying backward while standing. In everyday functional activities, overloading a muscle during the eccentric phase isn't nearly as common as overloading a muscle during the concentric phase; nevertheless, eccentric loading is a common cause of muscle strain injury. A muscle accustomed to eccentric loading is less likely to sustain an injury.

In addition to reducing the risk of injury, putting emphasis on eccentric contractions makes strength training more efficient. Muscles develop greater force (more tension is generated) by futilely trying to resist lengthening than by accomplishing shortening. Though a negative contraction is more efficient than a positive contraction (we can lower about 40 percent more resistance than we can lift), there's a greater risk of damaging muscle fibers through inflammation when performing negative contractions. For this reason, eccentric contractions must be performed with particular care—moderately slowly and with control.

Instruction

A full repetition is usually completed in six seconds. Perform the eccentric contraction at least twice as slowly as the concentric contraction. For example, during the bench press, alternate a four-second lowering phase with a two-second lifting phase.

Isometric Muscle Contraction

In weight-resistance yoga, force is mainly exerted using dynamic muscle action: moving a bony segment to pull a muscle's attachments closer together—concentric contraction—and moving a bony segment to separate a muscle's attachments—eccentric contraction. But with the third (and what I think is the oddest) kind of muscle contraction, there's no movement at all. Isometric, or static, contraction is tightening muscle without moving any bony segments. The force is exerted neither by overcoming resistance nor by being overcome by resistance. Tension is developed in muscles simply by squeezing them (e.g., contracting the chest without moving the arms) or by straining against immovable loads (e.g., contracting the chest by pushing outstretched arms against a wall).

The weight-resistance yoga regimen is composed of dynamic exercises because they're more effective than isometric exercises for increasing strength and mimicking everyday activities. Nevertheless, isometric contractions play valuable roles in the weight-resistance yoga regimen. They're used as a technique for increasing the maximal amount of weight that can be resisted.

Instruction

During the last repetition of a dynamic exercise, isometrically contract muscles whose function is to assist the muscles most involved. For example, at the end of a bench press, briefly hold the arms at or near the sticking point (with the help of a spotter to complete the repetition)

Isometric contractions are also used in exercises that work the stabilizing muscles, whose function is to hold bones still.

Instruction

Isometrically contract muscles whose primary function is stabilization. For example, to activate the multifidus, the critical inner-core spinal muscle, during the lower back extension exercise (lifting the trunk from a lying-face-down position), statically hold the extended position for two seconds after each concentric phase.

Most critically, isometric contractions play a key role in making weight-resistance yoga into a discipline of movement within stillness.

Stabilization

A muscle exerts equal force at its points of origin and insertion on bony segments, enabling both bony segments to move. Generally, though, one segment moves in such a way that it produces more favorable strengthening of the muscle. In order for the desired movement to occur in that segment, the other segment must be fixed—as must be the areas that radiate from it.

Take, for example, the biceps brachii, the two-headed muscle on the upper arm commonly called the biceps. The biceps brachii exerts equal force at its attachments on the shoulder blade and its attachments at the forearm (fig. 4.1). However, the origin at the shoulder weakly lifts the upper arm at the shoulder to the front (the anterior fibers of the deltoid and the upper fibers of the pectoralis major are the primary movers), while the insertion at the forearm strongly lifts the forearm at the elbow (the biceps brachii, along with the brachialis and brachioradialis, are the primary movers). (Indeed, by definition an attachment is considered as the origin exactly because it's the attachment that moves a bony segment less, and as the insertion because it's the attachment that moves a body segment more. The insertion is usually attached farther from the midline or center of the body.) So the more effective means of strengthening the biceps brachii is bending the elbow to move the forearm toward the shoulder.

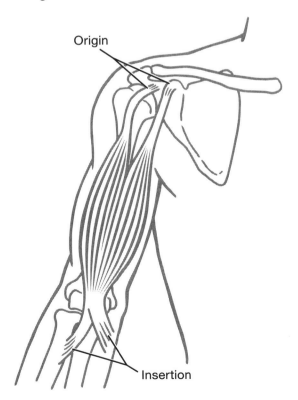

Fig. 4.1. Origin and insertion of biceps brachii

Nonmoving Stabilization

In order to effectively perform the standing barbell biceps curl, a common exercise for moving the forearm at the elbow joint by bending the elbow, the attachments of the biceps brachii at the shoulder joint must be stationary. This prevents the upper arm from moving forward and up, which would lessen the force of the action at the elbow. In fact, the entire shoulder complex must be fixed, or stabilized, in order to provide a base, or nonmoving body part, from which the biceps brachii can exert force on the forearm as it bends at the elbow.

This stabilization is accomplished by the static, or isometric, co-contraction of the muscles that perform shoulder joint flexion (the anterior fibers of the deltoid and upper fibers of the pectoralis major, assisted by smaller muscles, including the biceps brachii) and muscles that perform shoulder joint extension (posterior fibers of the deltoid, latissimus dorsi, teres major, and lower fibers of the pectoralis major). Ordinarily, an agonist group of muscles causes a specific movement (e.g., shoulder joint flexion), which is allowed by an antagonist group of muscles relaxing (e.g., shoulder joint extension). When both the agonist and antagonist muscles cooperate to stabilize—not move—the shoulder joint, the tendency to swing the upper arm forward (and sometimes swing it backward, as momentum takes hold) is inhibited: the upper arm is held at the side.

The wayward action at the shoulder joint to swing the upper arm up is often assisted by momentum initiated at the lower back. To inhibit the tendency to aid upper arm movement by swaying or lurching the lower back, the torso must be stabilized by the static contraction of the muscles that extend the lumbar spine (the erector spinae) and the muscles that flex the trunk (the muscles of the abdominal wall, especially the rectus abdominis). In addition, the tendency to bend and then straighten the legs to assist the thrusting moving of the spine must be inhibited by co-contracting the muscles that flex the hips (the iliopsoas) and knees (the hamstrings) and the muscles that extend the hips (the gluteus maximus) and knees (the quadriceps) (fig. 4.2).

Instruction

Performing the standing biceps curl without stabilizing the parts of the body that have a misguided inclination to assist the movement not only reduces the exercise's effectiveness (it subverts the assigned work of the targeted muscles by lessening their workload) but also increases the risk for injury. Invariably, a shoulder or lower back muscle will become injured. Keep the upper arms at the sides, the torso erect, and the legs straight.

Moving Stabilization

The accommodating nature of the shoulder blade (scapula), to which the upper arm connects, allows for a wide range of upper arm motion at the shoulder joint. But it seems to conflict with the upper arm's need for a stable base at the shoulder blade from which to exert force. How can the shoulder blade socket both promote optimal arm movement and also provide a stable base for arm movement? This dual function is accomplished by both tensing the shoulder blade muscles

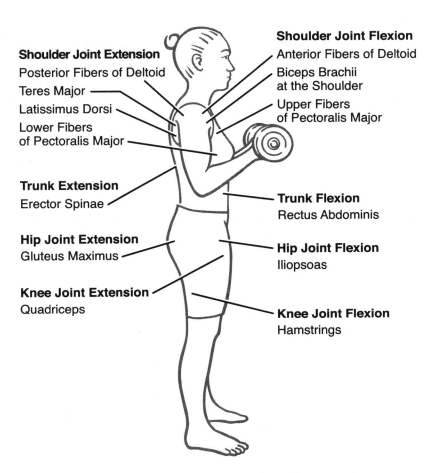

Shoulder Joint Extension
Posterior Fibers of Deltoid
Teres Major
Latissimus Dorsi
Lower Fibers
of Pectoralis Major

Shoulder Joint Flexion
Anterior Fibers of Deltoid
Biceps Brachii
at the Shoulder
Upper Fibers
of Pectoralis Major

Trunk Extension
Erector Spinae

Trunk Flexion
Rectus Abdominis

Hip Joint Extension
Gluteus Maximus

Hip Joint Flexion
Iliopsoas

Knee Joint Extension
Quadriceps

Knee Joint Flexion
Hamstrings

Fig. 4.2. Co-contraction of muscles in biceps curl

that release arm movement and also tensing (to a slightly lesser extent) the shoulder blade muscles that confine them. This process of producing tension in moving contralateral (opposing) muscles to meet the contradictory requirements of mobility and stabilization is called moving, or dynamic, stabilization.

Instruction

As the arms move first away from and then toward the body during shoulder joint pushing exercises (e.g., the shoulder press and bench press), and first toward and then away from the body during pulling exercises (e.g., the low row and lat pulldown), the shoulder blades (as well as the collar bone, or clavicle) move along with the arms. For example, during the shoulder press, for every three degrees of arm abduction, two degrees of raising the arm to the side and one degree of upwardly rotating the shoulder blade takes place. In order to stabilize as well as accommodate the arms reaching

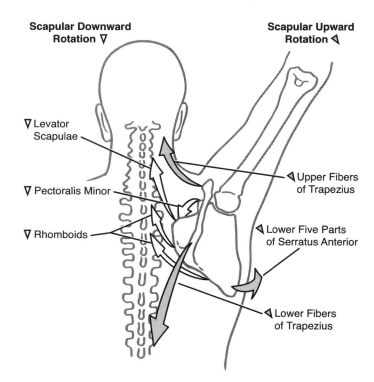

Scapular Downward Rotation ▽

Scapular Upward Rotation ◁

▽ Levator Scapulae

▽ Pectoralis Minor

▽ Rhomboids

◁ Upper Fibers of Trapezius

◁ Lower Five Parts of Serratus Anterior

◁ Lower Fibers of Trapezius

Fig. 4.3. Moving stabilization—direction of pull of shoulder blade muscles during arm abduction (The muscles that produce scapular upward rotation assist abduction of the arm, and the muscles that produce scapular downward rotation oppose abduction of the arm.)

out to the side, make slow, controlled movements of the shoulder blades by, in effect, attempting to downwardly rotate them as they rotate upward (fig. 4.3).

Weight-resistance yoga, like all hatha yoga, is a great simplification of life. It largely consists of a few rigid up-and-down or back-and-forth movements of the trunk, arms, and legs. But through being inordinately, stubbornly attentive to making these slight, nuanced, arduous movements of the trunk and limbs just so, while keeping the rest of the body essentially static, we find serenity.

5

GREAT EFFORT

Tapas

Like weight-surrender yoga's sustained stretching (which goes beyond our ordinary range of motion), weight-resistance yoga's intense strengthening (which goes beyond our ordinary production of force) demands great effort. Overcoming any tendencies toward distraction, drowsiness, and resignation, weight-resistance yogins carry out our exercises with *tapas,* burning desire.

Intensity

Any amount of weight load applied beyond normal will result in strength development. Setting the resistance to near maximal intensity, though, will elicit significantly greater and more efficient strength development than a lesser intensity. Intensity is defined by the maximal weight load for one repetition—the greatest amount we can lift once through the sticking point in the concentric, or positive, action of an exercise. Weight-resistance yogins perform exercises at a relatively high level of intensity: 80 to 85 percent of one repetition maximum. For example, if

the maximal load we can lift once is 100 pounds, the weight lifted for the set is about 80 or 85 pounds.

Due to differences in size and body structure, men are generally stronger than women. Men typically have more lean body mass and less fat, are heavier, have a taller and wider frame (which supports more muscle), and have broader shoulders (which provide greater leverage) than women. Although having less absolute strength than men (e.g., women have about 40 to 60 percent of men's upper-body strength), women are as capable as men of developing strength relative to their total muscle mass. So women, too, should lift weights at a high intensity.

Repetitions

The number of repetitions in a set is determined by whether the goal is to develop muscular strength or endurance or a mixture of both. Muscular strength is best developed by using heavier weights with few repetitions, and muscular endurance, by using lighter weights with many repetitions. Performing a set with 8 to 12 repetitions combines both muscular strength and endurance.

Instruction

The conventional wisdom is that lifting heavy weights makes you bulky. This notion, unsupported by science, is the reason why some who strength train, especially women, opt for performing strength exercises with lighter weights lifted many times. But in actuality, lifting a challenging weight load (80 to 85 percent of one repetition maximum) with few repetitions (sets of 8 repetitions) is more efficient for toning up (losing body fat) and slimming down (as long as you don't greatly increase your caloric consumption) than a light weight load with many repetitions. To burn more energy, use a regimen that includes more weight and fewer repetitions.

Speed

Each repetition should take at least six seconds, a moderate speed. This moderately slow velocity produces a higher level of muscle force than faster movement. While training at a fast velocity enhances explosive power, training at a moderate velocity enhances strength development. As movement speed decreases, muscle tension increases. So force production is higher at slower speeds. This longer time under tension not only results in more efficient strength gains but also is more conducive to training in a controlled manner.

Instruction

Perform an exercise at a moderately slow speed, usually six seconds. You should be able to stop the exercise at any point in the lifting or lowering movements. If you can't, you're moving too fast, and probably relying on momentum to assist the movement.

During free-weight (dumbbell and barbell), cable-and-pulley, and plate-loaded exercises, in which the resistance is constant, the muscle force produced to overcome the resistance varies according to the mechanical advantage of the joints involved. Consequently, the muscle force and resistance force aren't matched throughout the full range of motion. For example, during the dumbbell biceps curl, the most muscle force is exerted in the middle of the range of motion (a bell strength curve); during the leg curl, the most muscle force is exerted at the beginning of the range of motion (a descending strength curve); and during the bench press and squat, the most muscle force is exerted at the end of the range of motion (an ascending strength curve).

Instruction

To exert a constant maximal force throughout the full range of motion of an exercise, adjust the amount of force that's being applied by changing the speed. For example, gradually slow down as the muscle force becomes progressively less at the top range of the dumbbell biceps curl, between 90 and 135 degrees.

Range of Motion

A muscle becomes functionally stronger only in the movement location and range in which it encounters resistance. Moving a bony lever around its joint through a limited range of motion is easier on the muscles—especially if their sticking points are avoided—than moving it through a full range of motion (the degree of joint movement possible within the anatomic limitations of the joint structure). But full-range movements stimulate more muscle fibers, generating greater force.

Exercises in the Three Planes of Motion through a Full Range of Motion

For this reason, when possible and safe, the weight-resistance yoga protocol requires that when bones are being worked in any of the three possible planes of motion (the antero-posterior or sagittal plane, where front to back movements take place; the lateral or frontal plane, where side to side movements take place; and the transverse or horizontal plane, where rotational movements take place—the three general locations where the great variety of bodily movements takes place), they should be moved through a full range of motion. For example, at the shoulder joint, optimal flexion of the humerus occurs in the anterior-posterior plane (lifting the arm up in front) to 170 to 180 degrees (fig. 5.1); at the hip joint, optimal abduction of the femur occurs in the lateral plane (moving the leg out to the

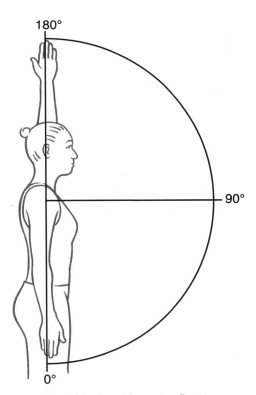

Fig. 5.1. Shoulder joint flexion

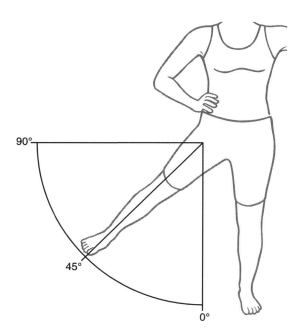

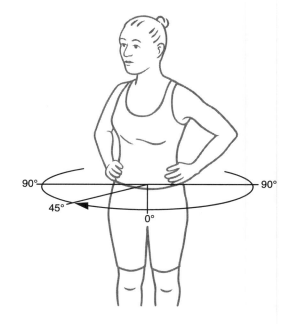

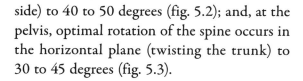

Fig. 5.2. Hip joint abduction   Fig. 5.3. Lumbar spine rotation

side) to 40 to 50 degrees (fig. 5.2); and, at the pelvis, optimal rotation of the spine occurs in the horizontal plane (twisting the trunk) to 30 to 45 degrees (fig. 5.3).

Beginning Point

There's an optimal length at which muscle fibers generate maximal force during an exercise. Contracting a muscle at its optimal length applies not only to where the movement of a bony segment is completed but also to where it is initiated.

Instruction

To increase the distance over which force can be generated, pre-stretch targeted muscles before contracting them. For example, when beginning the machine chest fly, pull the shoulders back

to stretch the pectoral muscles before contracting them (fig. 5.4). But don't force muscles beyond their limits when in the stretched position. Instead, gradually increase your range of motion over several weeks or even months.

Strengthening muscles through their full range of motion also has another benefit: stretching opposing muscles. When muscles are contracted through a wide range of motion, their opposing muscles are relaxed through a wide range of motion.

Instruction

By pairing exercises for opposing muscle groups, you increase and maintain not only joint strength but joint flexibility, as well.

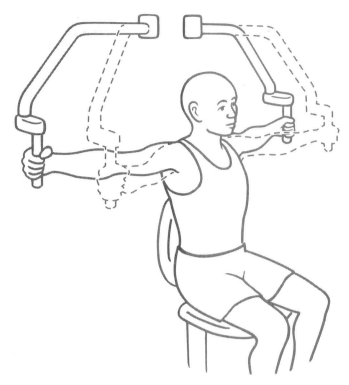

Fig. 5.4. Pre-stretch in machine chest fly

The Sticking Point

The movements produced by muscle contractions must go past the sticking point, the weakest point in the range of motion, where movement might stall. For example, a common sticking point in the bench press is the midpoint, where the front deltoids are involved less and the pectorals and triceps are involved more.

Contractions that don't challenge the sticking point by moving through a wide range of motion are barely worth performing.

The Midpoint

Locking your elbows or knees during a strengthening exercise may cause excessive pressure on their joints. Although perhaps no harm will be done if explosive locking is avoided (by fully straightening the elbows and knees gradually and with control), the compression forces that result from locking joints are so great that it's safer to keep the elbow and knee joints slightly bent in the top position of an exercise.

Exceptions to this rule are the knee extension and the front arm raise, during which the legs and arms, respectively, can be brought up to ninety degrees and momentarily locked because the leverage isn't straight up and down (i.e., the weight isn't traveling straight down through the joints).

Even when it's safe, however, locking

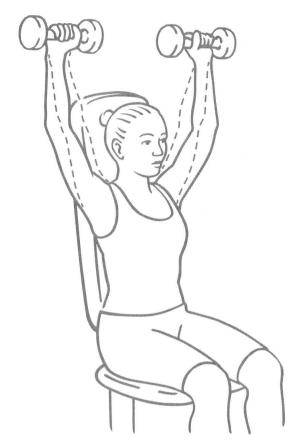

Fig. 5.5. Keeping elbows bent in 90-to-135-degree shoulder press

joints is inefficient. Leaving a little slack in a joint that's being moved increases the time a muscle is under tension; the more tension is produced, the more efficient the exercise is in enhancing strength development.

Instruction

During lower-body exercises, such as squats and leg presses, and upper-body exercises, such as bench and shoulder presses, keep some play in the knees and elbows, respectively (fig. 5.5).

The End Point

At the end of the eccentric, or negative, contraction phase of a repetition, there's a tendency to bring the moving bony segment all the way to the resting position and begin the next repetition by thrusting or yanking the weight using momentum.

Instruction

Don't trespass beyond the starting position (an inch or so from the resting position) until the set is over.

It's equally important at the end of the eccentric contraction phase of the repetition to avoid the tendency to bring the moving bony segment to less than the starting position. A muscle performs more concentrically loaded work if it's fully stretched (eccentrically loaded) just before shortening, creating a stretch-shortening cycle. Like a spring being stretched, elastic components of the muscle and tendon that are elongated during the eccentric action store energy—which is released during the concentric action as the elastic components, like a stretched spring when the tension is taken off, return to their resting length.

Instruction
Gradually build up tolerance to near maximal stretching during the eccentric action.

To prevent injury, however, sometimes the range of motion of an exercise should be restricted, especially for those who are beginning strength training. For example, raising the arms past ninety degrees during the eccentric phase of the lat pulldown—a latissimus dorsi (the broad back muscle) exercise that incorporates a powerful, repetitive arm motion—risks an impingement injury (tendonitis of the supraspinatus, a rotator cuff muscle). It's better to sacrifice full range of motion by keeping the shoulders down and the upper arms at shoulder level before bringing the upper arms back and down toward the sides (fig. 5.6).

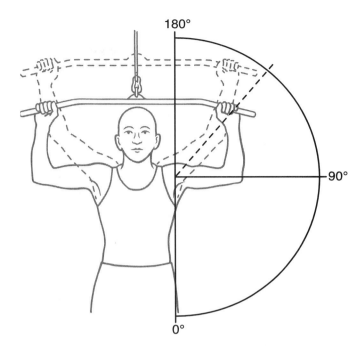

Fig. 5.6. Lat pulldown correct starting position (and ending position for eccentric phase)

Muscle Exhaustion

Muscle exhaustion (temporary fatigue or volitional failure) is the point in a set when a muscle can no longer contract concentrically to overcome resistance. This is a good thing. Strength is only fully developed by fatiguing targeted muscles, whether over a long set with many repetitions or a short set with few repetitions.

Muscle exhaustion is most efficiently attained by stressing the anaerobic energy system, which produces ATP (adenosine triphosphate, the substance in a cell that provides energy for muscle fibers to contract and thereby to exert force) without oxygen during a burst of intense physical activity. We can safely achieve muscle exhaustion within the short-duration (about 1.5 minutes) time frame of the anaerobic pathways by performing 8 to 12 repetitions at a moderate movement speed (about 6 or 7 seconds per repetition) with approximately 80 to 85 percent of maximum resistance (heavy enough to provide a high-strength stimulus and light enough to avoid injury).

Instruction

If you resist less weight than 80 percent of your maximum for 8 to 12 repetitions, you'll benefit less. You know you're using the most efficient weight load when you can perform your predetermined number of repetitions to muscle exhaustion—that is, until no further repetitions can be completed using proper technique.

Remember to maintain good form, especially as you approach muscle exhaustion, when you might be tempted to push on to meet your repetition goal. Recklessly propelling weights that are too heavy leads to injury. If you can meet your goal only by using poor form, lower the workload. If you can exceed your repetition goal, increase the workload.

The Gaze

Because sense withdrawal in weight-resistance yoga doesn't entail closing off the sense organs, we keep our eyes open during each set—but cease reacting to impressions around us. Instead of alertly looking from place to place, we gaze at a single place.

Instruction

When your head is immobile during an exercise, focus your eyes on a place in the medium distance. When your head moves, focus on a narrow path. Looking with a fixed focus inhibits mindless habituation in which you vacantly go through the motions of the exercise. By constantly fixing your attention on a specific place, you also shut out what is alluring or intrusive in your everyday life. You direct your attention within.

Breathing

Weight-resistance training is essentially a discipline with a bipolar dynamic. The opposing forces are types of muscle movement (each exercise consists of concentric and eccentric contractions) or of bone movement (each exercise consists of actions that move a bony part away from and toward the body—more specifically, that pull a bone away from the center of its joint and toward the center of its joint). Which is why, unlike the ungainly matching of rhythmic breathing to asana movements (first applied in the 1920s to make the conditioning asanas competitive with gymnastics exercises), rhythmic breathing is perfectly matched to the bipolar movements of strength training. Take, for example, the standing biceps curl and the triceps pull-down exercises.

To perform the biceps curl, the three elbow flexors (biceps brachii, brachialis, and brachioradialis) contract to move the forearm toward the shoulder by bending the elbow. We breathe in during the upward movement of the forearm toward the chest and breathe out during the forearm's movement down and away from chest.

To perform the triceps extension, the elbow extensors (the three heads of triceps brachii) contract to move the forearm away from the shoulder by straightening the elbow. We breathe out during the forearm's downward movement and breathe in during the forearm's upward movement.

Deep Breathing

The primary source of energy to muscles during a weight-resistance yoga exercise—a short-duration, high-intensity exercise—is anaerobic energy production: energy production without the immediate need for oxygen. The reason for increased difficulty of breathing, manifested by a heaving chest and gasping breath, during the last few repetitions of a set is that the respiratory and circulatory systems are desperately attempting to meet the sudden increased demand for oxygen in the muscles.

Instruction

You can avoid the gasping for breath during the last few repetitions by breathing deeply and evenly from the start. Deep, even, and continuous diaphragmatic breathing allows you to take control of the wild breath.

Perform deep diaphragmatic breathing as follows.

Inhalation: Inhalation is the drawing of air into the lungs during breathing.

Instruction

Inhale before initiating movement and on the release of effort (e.g., when you lower a weight). As the air enters the top portion of the lungs, push the diaphragm down on the abdomen, letting the belly expand slightly. As the air moves into the middle portion of the lungs, expand the middle and lower ribs. As the air moves into the lower portion of the lungs, complete the inhalation by filling the lungs in the front, sides, and back, relaxing the belly as much as possible. (The dimension of deep breathing often neglected is the sideways expansion of the intercostals, the muscles between the ribs.)

Exhalation: Exhalation is the expelling of air from the lungs during breathing.

Instruction

Exhale on exertion (e.g., when you lift a weight). Exhalation is ordinarily passive. But during weight-resistance yoga, as the chest muscles and diaphragm relax and the ribs move in and close together, contract the abdomen to expel the air.

Nasal Breathing

Ordinarily, nasal breathing, performed with a closed mouth, facilitates diaphragmatic breathing. During the forced breathing of strenuous exercise, however, nasal breathing is difficult to maintain. For this reason, it's considered an advanced technique.

Instruction

Breathe through your nose. If inhaling and exhaling through your nose isn't possible or is extremely difficult, inhale through your mouth and exhale through your nose.

Continuous Breathing

Performing high-intensity resistance exercises temporarily increases blood pressure. This increase isn't harmful. Blood pressure returns to normal when the body is at rest. Holding the breath during a strengthening exercise, however, is potentially dangerous. It may cause light-headedness by limiting blood flow to the head and may cause a severe increase in blood pressure by limiting blood return to the heart.

Instruction

To prevent constricted blood flow and elevated blood pressure, breathe evenly and continuously during each exercise repetition, inhaling during negative muscle contractions and exhaling during positive muscle contractions (e.g., during the standing biceps curl, exhale during the lifting movement and inhale during the lowering movement).

During the weight-resistance yoga session, we transcend our everyday existence by refusing to conform to its most elementary tendencies. The most important of these refusals, yoga scholar Mircea Eliade argues, is the regulation of the breath—"the 'refusal' to breathe like the majority of mankind, that is, non-rhythmically."[1] "Through *pranayama* [yogic breathing]," Eliade elaborates, "the yogin seeks to attain direct knowledge of the pulsation of his own life, the organic energy discharged by inhalation and exhalation."[2]

Although many styles of strength training recommend coordinating the exhalation and inhalation of the breath with the respective contraction and elongation of the muscles of the limbs and trunk, in weight-resistance yoga it sometimes feels as if the rhythmic movements are faithfully serving the breath. Making the breath slow, deep, nasal, and even—which is nothing less than knowing through action the very essence of life—facilitates a state of calm that's largely inaccessible to us in our everyday existence.

6

ACCORD AND ACCEPTANCE

Over the course of six months of four daily workout routines per week, a number of exercise determinants are brought into accord with one another in order to establish a weight-resistance yoga regimen that can be performed more or less for the rest of our lives. (The exact make up of this regimen is contingent on several factors—the most critical being the age, training experience, fitness, health, and goals of the individual developing the regimen.)

Daily Exercise Routine Determinants

Selection of Exercises

The capacity for movement of the body's bones differs greatly. Joints allow or limit the movement of variously sized and shaped bones. In some joints, several different directions of movement are possible. In others, only a few directions of movement are possible. In yet others, no movement at all is possible. The strengthening exercises of weight-resistance yoga are determined by the movement capabilities of the major joints. Take, for example, those of the shoulder and hip joints. Both are freely movable joints enclosed by capsules that

secrete fluid to lubricate the ends of the bones that form the joints.

The upper arm bone, the humerus, with its ball-shaped end that fits into the shallow socket of the joint, can be moved in eight basic directions (flexion, extension, adduction, abduction, horizontal adduction, horizontal abduction, internal rotation, and external rotation), with much variation in position and range. Allowing for combined movements, the shoulder joint needs six exercises per upper-body routine to match all the directions.

The hip joint, also a ball-and-socket joint, has a thicker and denser capsule, which favors leg stability over mobility. The upper leg bone, the femur, moves in six directions (flexion, extension, adduction, abduction, internal rotation, and external rotation), with little possibility for variation. Allowing for combined movements, the hip joint needs only four exercises per lower-body routine.

Through systematically examining all the movements of the major joints in this manner, the number and type of strengthening exercises has been determined for the weight-resistance yoga routines.

Number of Sets of Exercises

To develop muscle mass (usually for the glamour muscles), weight lifters commonly perform each exercise three times per daily routine. Unconcerned with bulk, weight-resistance yogins perform each exercise only once per daily routine. One set performed with great effort is sufficient to develop and maintain a suitable level of strength.

Series of Exercises

Weight lifters don't usually bother performing exercises to strengthen (what they consider to be) the dreary muscles of the neck, shoulder blades, spine, hips, and shins. Weight-resistance yogins, in contrast, are systematically, comprehensively inclusive. In order to strengthen the muscles that produce all the major joint movements, we perform a great variety of exercises during the week. Approximately fifteen separate exercises are performed per daily routine (performing an exercise only once per daily routine allows for the time to perform this number), totaling approximately sixty different exercises in a week with four daily workout routines.

Each daily routine is composed of a series of exercises that revolve around a different joint. Exercises within each series might work on slightly or totally different planes of motion or might complete a range of motion. The upper-body routine consists of three series: for the shoulder joint (about six exercises), elbow joint (two exercises), and shoulder girdle (four exercises). The lower-body routine consists of four series: for the trunk (four exercises for the lumbar spine and four exercises for the cervical spine*), hip joint (four exercises), knee joint (two exercises), and ankle joint (three exercises). (See the sample exercise routines below beginning on page 51.)

Sequence of Exercises

The order of the exercises is determined by two physiological principles. The first principle is that muscle groups fatigue as they strengthen. For this reason, we perform the most-demanding exercises before the least-demanding exercises. When targeting the same muscle group, we first perform large muscle, single joint exercises (e.g., the chest fly, which works the pectoralis major). We next perform large muscle, multiple joint exercises (e.g., the chest press, which works the fatigued pectoralis major with the assistance of the fresh triceps brachii). And we last perform small muscle, single joint exercises (e.g., the dumbbell kickback, which works the triceps brachii). If small, assisting muscles are fatigued first, we're forced to complete large muscle, multiple joint exercises with less than full capability, which risks injury.

The second principle is that skeletal muscles or muscle groups are related in agonist/antagonist pairs located on opposite sides of a joint. Despite their names, agonists and antagonists act in conjunction. Although they may act to prevent movement, these pairs generally work together to move a bony segment. For example, when the elbow flexion muscles

---

*Cervical spine exercises may actually be performed as part of an upper- or lower-body routine. See Addenda to the Day Two Lower-Body Routine and Cervical Spine Exercises table on page 54.

(biceps brachii, brachialis, and brachioradialis)—acting as the agonist—shorten and contract to "close" a straightened elbow joint, the elbow extension muscle (triceps brachii)—acting as the antagonist—lengthens and relaxes. And when the elbow extension muscle—acting as the agonist—shortens and contracts to "open" a bent elbow joint, the elbow flexion muscles—acting as the antagonist—lengthen and relax. To maintain musculoskeletal balance, we must strengthen both muscles or muscle groups of an agonist/antagonist muscle pair.

We cannot maintain musculo-skeletal balance, however, unless it's already present. Before embarking on a program of balanced strengthening exercises, weight-resistance yogins make certain that our skeleton is structurally balanced in the first place—that our posture is standard (i.e., optimal). To assess our posture and, if necessary, to receive a prescribed treatment plan of exercises to correct our posture, we must turn to a weight-resistance yoga teacher, physical therapist, doctor, or other expert in posture. An effective treatment plan for defective posture consists of both strength and flexibility exercises.

Remedial Exercises to Improve Posture

The key to structural balance of the skeleton is having equal pull by muscles located on opposite sides of a joint. An imbalance in these forces affects range of motion, resulting in loss of mobility. Muscle imbalance is often due to overly lengthened (weak) muscles and overly shortened (tight) muscles. Lengthening and shortening of our muscles occur as a result of our body adapting to long periods of time spent in a misaligned posture—sitting, standing, or walking with habitually faulty posture.

Consider, for example, someone with the mildly stooped posture that includes a jutting neck; splayed shoulder blades (the scapulae pulled away from the spine and downwardly rotated); hunched upper back (the thoracic spine with an increased posterior curve); abdomen scrunched up, coupled with lower-back muscles flattened (the pelvis rotated posteriorly); and bent hips, knees, and ankles. When habitual, these postural faults strain the neck, causing headaches; elongate the middle and lower trapezius (a mighty shoulder girdle muscle), diminishing its ability to assist arm elevation; reduce the mobility of the thoracic cavity, restricting the lungs and making breathing difficult; strain the lower back muscles, resulting in lumbar back pain; and tighten the legs, causing cramps.

The customary weight-resistance yoga regimen, which consists of paired exercises that strengthen opposing muscles (agonists and antagonists) would partly exacerbate the imbalance: overly lengthened muscles would be shortened, but overly shortened muscles would be further shortened. The customary weight-surrender yoga regime, which consists of paired counter poses that stretch opposing muscles, would lengthen overly shortened muscles but would further lengthen overly lengthened muscles. So it, too, would partly exacerbate the imbalance. Therefore, a temporary postural program is put in place (under the advisement of an expert) consisting of weight-resistance yoga exercises that strengthen overly lengthened muscles (in a state of prolonged elongation) without the usual opposing exercises, and weight-surrender yoga postures that stretch overly shortened muscles (in a state of prolonged contraction) without the usual counter poses.

Take, for example, the misalignment caused by the jutting neck, one of the imbalances of the person described above. The muscles of the neck support the head, which can weigh about fifteen pounds. A head that's protruding forward strains neck and back muscles. To compensate for the downward line of vision, the head is tilted up. As a consequence, the posterior neck muscles are overly shortened, and the anterior neck muscles are overly lengthened.

To strengthen the overly elongated anterior muscles, the person might perform the cervical flexion exercise, which is movement of the head toward the chest (fig. 6.1) (without practicing the opposing exercise, extension). This cervical strengthening exercise could be supplemented by two stretching poses: the Hare Pose, which includes tucking the chin in toward the chest and placing the head on the floor in front of the knees, to stretch the overly shortened posterior neck muscles (fig. 6.2) (without practicing a counter pose, such as the Bow), and the Mountain Pose, which includes lifting up the head while the chin is parallel to the floor, allowing the entire neck to release (fig. 6.3).

In this manner, all the misaligned areas are addressed until the optimal length/tension relationship for muscles is restored throughout the body. The body is, in effect, reeducated.

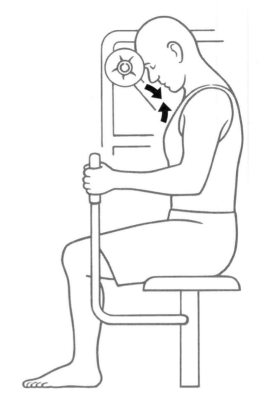

Fig. 6.1. Cervical flexion exercise for strengthening overly elongated anterior neck muscles

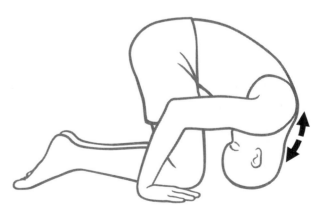

Fig. 6.2. Hare Pose for stretching overly shortened posterior neck muscles

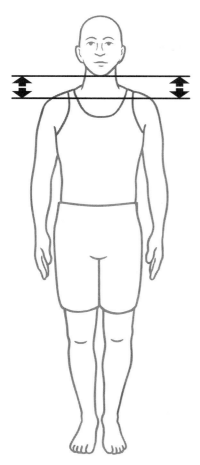

Fig. 6.3. Mountain Pose for releasing anterior
and posterior neck muscles

Once proper posture is achieved, the customary weight-resistance yoga and weight-surrender yoga routines, with their familiar protocols of complementary exercises, are initiated to maintain balance at the joints.

It's difficult to maintain balanced posture throughout the day. Most of us tend to lapse. Bent over at our desk or in our driver's seat, we give in to the pull of gravity, letting our bones become somewhat misaligned. By performing regular weight-resistance yoga and weight-surrender yoga exercise routines, we systematically work muscles in order to bring misaligned bones back into their proper place. In this way, we continually restore standard posture before a slight, temporary musculo-skeletal imbalance settles into a stubborn, habitual imbalance.

Practice Time of Exercises

There's no best time to practice weight-resistance yoga. It's is a matter of personal preference and availability. Nevertheless, weight-resistance yoga training, which maintains or increases muscular strength and endurance, must be compatible with training to maintain or increase the two other components of fitness: flexibility (in the form of weight-surrender yoga) and cardiorespiratory capacity.

Flexibility

If weight-resistance yoga and weight-surrender yoga are performed back to back, weight-resistance yoga should be performed first. Either one of these disciplines can be performed in the morning and the other in the evening of the same day. They can be performed on alternating days.

Cardiorespiratory Activity

An elevated heart rate isn't a direct indicator of an aerobic training experience. Weight-resistance training, which elevates the heart rate, doesn't increase aerobic capacity—not even in the form of circuit weight training, which involves moving quickly from machine to machine to perform sets. To effectively improve cardiorespiratory endurance, an exercise must rhythmically utilize large-muscle groups, the most convenient of which are those of the lower body, for a minimum sustained period (at least 20 to 30 minutes) at a moderate to high intensity (between 40 and 85 percent of maximum capacity).

Strength training does, however, offer benefits to those who perform daily activities and exercises that elevate the cardiorespiratory system. Take long-distance running. Weight resistance increases muscular strength and endurance to aid running economy and durability, facilitates breathing by improving posture, and lowers the risk of injuries at joints by strengthening connective tissue and bone.

Performing a high-intensity lower-body strength-training workout before a cardiorespiratory workout, which usually involves strenuously moving the legs, may compromise the cardiorespiratory activity: localized spine, hip, knee, and ankle muscle fatigue may cause sluggishness and susceptibility to injury. Conversely, the muscle fatigue that results from cardiovascular endurance training performed before lower-body strength training may prevent peak strength performance and risks an overuse injury.

Instruction

When feasible, perform cardiorespiratory endurance training and lower-body strength training on different days. If this isn't possible, simply choose the order that fits your primary goal. If your primary goal is to improve the functions of the heart and lungs and maximize weight loss, then endurance training should be performed first. If toning lower-body muscles is your primary goal, then strength training should precede endurance conditioning.

The Weekly Exercise Routine

To activate different muscle fibers, weight lifters commonly perform variations of strengthening exercises for a few glamorous muscle groups. For example, they might stack three or four exercises for the "pecs" (such as cable flies, push-ups, and bench presses) or "lats" (lat pulldowns, seated low rows, and bent-over rows). Weight-resistance yogins perform no more than two exercises for any given part of the body in a daily routine.

Variations of Exercises

Weight-resistance yogins do, however, recognize the importance of activating different muscle fibers. So we, too, perform a number of variations of exercises for a targeted muscle group—spread out over four (or possibly five) routines per week.

Varying an exercise for a targeted muscle group can be accomplished in two ways: by performing exercises that either change the motion while using the same or different types of equipment, or keep the same or very similar motion while changing the type of equipment.

Variations in Motion

Variations in motion can be achieved by performing exercises that change the following:

The angle of motion—for example, the incline bench press, which recruits more of the chest muscles that originate at the collar bone, by moving the arms in front at a 130-degree angle from their resting position while standing; and the decline bench press, which recruits more of the chest muscles that originate at the first six ribs and sternum by moving the arms in front at a 60-degree angle from their resting position while standing (fig. 6.4).

The range of motion—for example, the 0-to-90-degree front dumbbell raise, which moves the arms in front in a 0-to-90-degree arc from the thighs to the shoulders; and the 90-to-180-degree front dumbbell raise, using a lighter weight, which moves the arms in front in a 90-to-180-degree arc from the shoulders to overhead (see fig. 6.5 on page 46).

The plane of motion—for example, the wide lat pulldown, which engages the upper lats to adduct the arms, and the seated low row, which engages the lower lats to extend the arms (see fig. 6.6 on page 46).

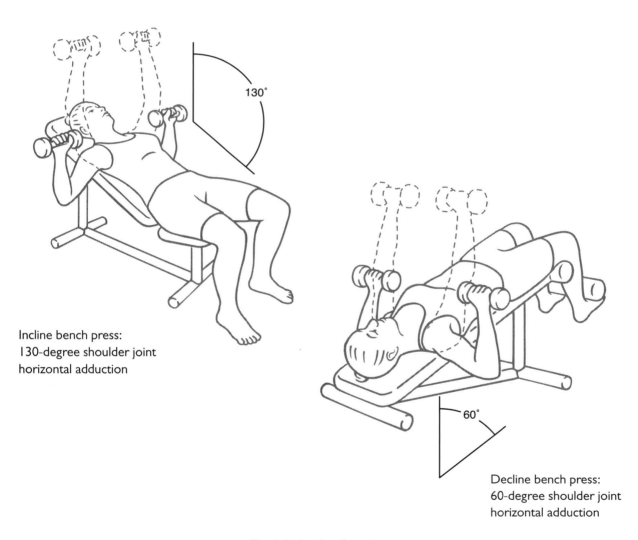

Incline bench press:
130-degree shoulder joint
horizontal adduction

Decline bench press:
60-degree shoulder joint
horizontal adduction

Fig. 6.4. Angle of motion

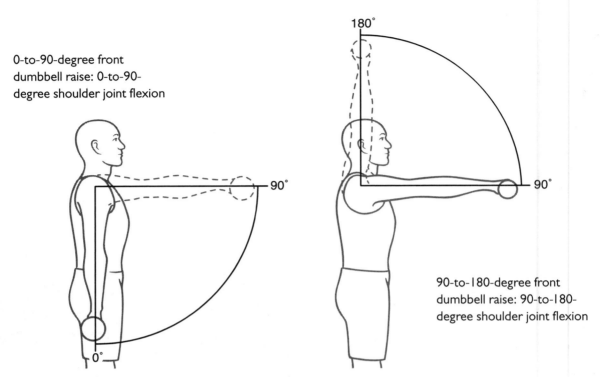

0-to-90-degree front dumbbell raise: 0-to-90-degree shoulder joint flexion

180°

90°

0°

90-to-180-degree front dumbbell raise: 90-to-180-degree shoulder joint flexion

Fig. 6.5. Range of motion

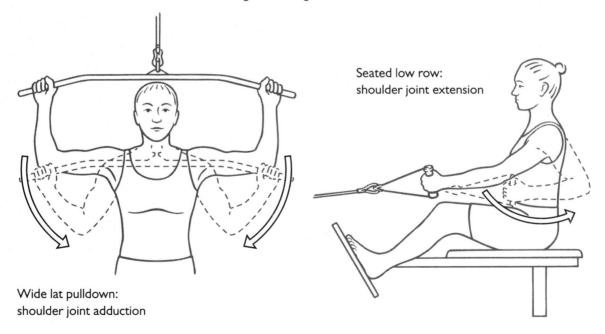

Seated low row: shoulder joint extension

Wide lat pulldown: shoulder joint adduction

Fig. 6.6. Plane of motion

The pattern of motion—either rotary, which involves curved movement for one joint action, or linear, which involves straight movement for two or more joint actions. For example, the chest cable crossover fly, a rotary exercise in which only the pectoralis major muscle at the shoulder joints produces movement; and the chest press, a linear exercise in which the triceps muscle at the elbow joints assist the pectoralis major muscle to produce movement (fig. 6.7); or the knee extension, a rotary exercise in which only the quadriceps muscles at the knee joints produce movement; and the leg press, a linear exercise in which the hamstrings (upper fibers) and gluteus maximus muscles at the hip joints assist the quadriceps muscles to produce movement (see fig. 6.8 on page 48).

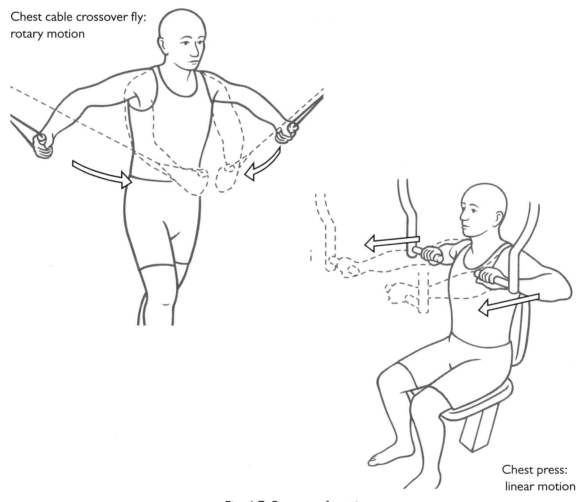

Chest cable crossover fly: rotary motion

Chest press: linear motion

Fig. 6.7. Pattern of motion

Knee extension: rotary motion

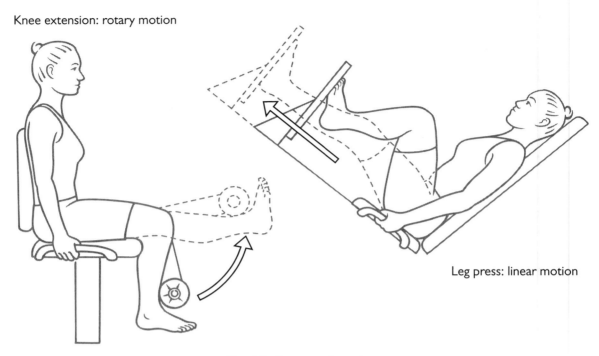

Leg press: linear motion

Fig. 6.8. Pattern of motion

Variations in Equipment

Variations in equipment can be achieved by performing exercises that use the following:

Free weights—which develop force by using a constant weight load to oppose gravitational resistance (fig. 6.9).

Cable-and-pulley machines—which develop force by using a constant weight load to oppose mechanical resistance (fig. 6.10).

Lever-arm-and-cam machines—which develop force by using a variable weight load to oppose mechanical resistance (fig. 6.11).

Two other types of equipment, plate-loaded machines and calisthenics apparatus, share characteristics with these three basic types. Plate-loaded machines are similar to free weights (the weight is constant) and to lever-arm-and-cam machines (the movement trajectory against mechanical resistance is prescribed). Calisthenics apparatus are similar to free weights (the weight is constant, and freedom of movement is allowed against gravitational resistance).

Each of the three basic types of equipment—free weights, cable-and-pulley machines, and lever-arm-and-cam machines—has its advantages and disadvantages.

The Advantage of
Free Weights over Machines

Free weights (dumbbells and barbells) provide constant resistance that allows for a change of direction of movement. This is in contrast to lever-arm-and-cam machines, which

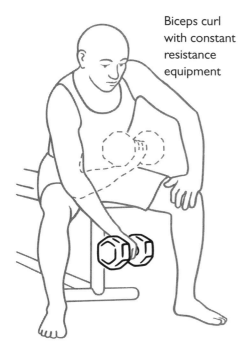

Biceps curl with constant resistance equipment

Fig. 6.9. Free weights

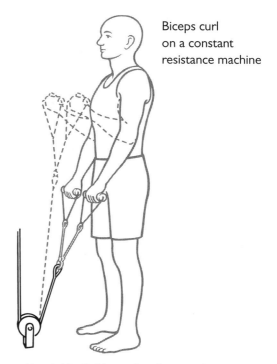

Biceps curl on a constant resistance machine

Fig. 6.10. Cable-and-pulley machine

force movement along a predetermined track, but similar to cable-and-pulley machines. However, unlike both kinds of machines, which provide external stabilization, free weights provide little or no external stabilization; so free-weight exercises require us to provide our own stabilization.

As a result, free-weight exercises incorporate more of the skills we need to perform the strengthening activities of daily life. Unlike the machine chest press, for example, the bench press, which uses a barbell, calls on our proprioception (sensing joint position and joint movement), balance (maintaining the body's center of gravity over the base of support), and coordination (performing smooth, accurate, and controlled movements of targeted muscles with the assistance

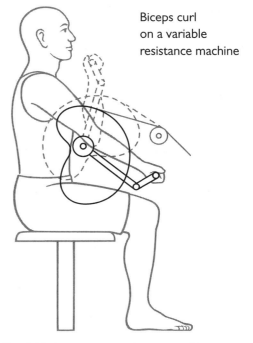

Biceps curl on a variable resistance machine

Fig. 6.11. Lever-arm-and-cam machine

of helping and stabilizing muscles) to attain stabilization.

The Advantage of Machines over Free Weights

In contrast to free-weight exercises, which sometimes can't easily provide resistance directly opposed to gravity, machines can always provide an efficient and optimal direction of resistance. For example, to perform a lat pulldown with free weights, we'd have to hang upside down and pull a barbell upward toward our shoulders. It's much more practical (and safer) to pull a bar or handles down using a lat pulldown machine.

The Advantage of Free Weights and Constant-Resistance Machines over Variable-Resistance Machines

Free weights and cable-and-pulley machines (which are mechanically similar to free weights) can provide freedom of movement that lever-arm-and-cam machines usually can't. Free-weight and cable-and-pulley-machine exercises allow for multiple actions of the muscles most involved. For example, in order to fully work the gluteus maximus, which extends and externally rotates the hip, a gluteus maximus cable-and-pulley-machine exercise can incorporate both bringing the buttock and upper posterior thigh backward and rotating them outward.

The Advantage of Variable-Resistance Machines over Free Weights and Constant-Resistance Machines

By providing variable resistance, lever-arm-and-cam machines do a reasonable (but not perfect) job of matching up the muscle force and resistance force more efficiently than do free weights and cable-and-pulley machines. Compare, for example, the supine dumbbell fly and the pec dec fly, which both target the pectoralis major. In the supine dumbbell fly, the resistance against gravity is greatest at the beginning position, when the arms are spread out and the pectoralis major muscle is least engaged; the resistance against gravity is least in the midpoint, when the arms are straight up and the pectoralis major muscle is fully engaged. This is a poor matching of muscle force and resistance force. In the pec dec fly, in contrast, the machine's resistance is lowest at the beginning and highest at the midpoint, which matches the recruitment of the pectoralis major muscle fibers.

A strength-training program should include both constant and variable resistance, mixing free-weight and machine exercises. Beginners, however, should consider using lever-arm-and-cam machines and cable-and-pulley machines instead of free weights (especially for exercises in which the muscle force and resistance force don't match up) because they provide more stability and safety.

A Sample
Weekly Exercise Routine

An effective, efficient, and safe weekly routine is composed of daily routines that work muscle groups in pairs (to achieve balanced joint strength) and from most difficult to least difficult (to avoid fatiguing assisting muscles). Over the course of the week, all the major muscles of the body are worked at least two times. A common weekly sequencing to achieve this goal alternates upper-body and lower-body exercises for four days.

Recovery Time for Daily Routines

Recovery (and adaptation) time for a workout is the rest period between successive workouts. Rest is needed in order for the targeted muscle group to refill its store of glycogen (the carbohydrate energy source in muscles) depleted during strength training.

Instruction

Allow one complete day of recovery between successive similar workouts. If you perform full-body exercises on day one, rest the next day, and wait until day three to perform them again. If you perform upper-body exercises on day one, wait until day three to perform them again. You may, however, perform lower-body exercises on day two.

Because the three types of equipment have their advantages and disadvantages, each type of equipment is used systematically during the week. Three daily upper-body routines solely or prominently consist of lever-arm-and-cam machines, cable-and-pulley machines, or free weights. (These three upper-body routines may be rotated over three weeks, or all three may be performed in one week by adding an extra workout.) Two daily lower-body routines prominently consist of lever-arm-and-cam machines or cable-and-pulley machines.

By practicing exercises in this orderly manner over the course of a week—assigning different but related exercise routines to each of the four sessions—the possible variations in a weekly strength-training practice are brought into accord.

On the following pages are exercise tables (with complete information) for one upper-body routine and one lower-body routine and exercise lists (with partial information) for two more upper-body routines and one more lower-body routine.

DAY ONE

Upper-Body Routine
Using Cable-and-Pulley Machines

	First Pair	Second Pair	Third Pair	Fourth Pair	Fifth Pair	Sixth Pair
Joint	Shoulder joint	Shoulder joint	Shoulder joint	Elbow joint	Shoulder girdle	Shoulder girdle
Exercise	Lat pulldown	High row	Seated low row	Biceps curl	Shoulder pulldown	Shoulder diagonal pulldown
Movement	Shoulder joint adduction (upper arm downward movement from side)	Shoulder joint horizontal abduction (upper arm horizontal movement away from chest)	Shoulder joint extension (upper arm movement straight back)	Elbow joint flexion (forearm movement toward shoulder by bending elbow)	Shoulder girdle depression (shoulder blade downward movement)	Shoulder girdle adduction (shoulder blade backward movement)
Muscle Most Involved	Latissimus dorsi (upper fibers)	Infraspinatus	Latissimus dorsi (lower fibers)	Biceps brachii	Trapezius (lower fibers)	Rhomboids
Equipment	C-P lat pulldown machine	D C-S P machine	C-P row machine	D C-S P machine	C-P lat pulldown machine	D C-S P machine
Joint	Shoulder joint	Shoulder joint	Shoulder joint	Elbow joint	Shoulder girdle	Shoulder girdle
Exercise	Shoulder press	Cable crossover fly	Front raise	Triceps pushdown	Shoulder shrug	Scaption raise
Movement	Shoulder joint abduction (upper arm upward movement out to side)	Shoulder joint horizontal adduction (upper arm horizontal movement toward chest)	Shoulder joint flexion (arm movement straight forward)	Elbow joint extension (forearm movement away from shoulder by straightening elbow)	Shoulder girdle elevation (shoulder blade upward movement)	Shoulder girdle abduction (shoulder blade forward movement)
Muscle Most Involved	Deltoid (middle fibers)	Pectoralis major	Deltoid (anterior fibers)	Triceps brachii	Trapezius (middle fibers)	Serratus anterior
Equipment	C-P crossover machine	C-P crossover machine	C-P crossover machine	C-P triceps machine	D C-S P machine	C-P crossover machine

Key: C-P = cable-and-pulley; D C-S P = dual cable-and-swivel pulley

DAY TWO
Lower-Body Routine
Featuring Lever-Arm-and-Cam Machines
and Plate-Loaded Machines

	First Pair	Second Pair	Third Pair	Fourth Pair	Fifth Pair	Sixth Pair
Joint	Trunk	Trunk	Hip joint	Hip joint	Knee joint	Ankle joint
Exercise	Back raise	Side bend	Bent-Leg Hip Extension	Hip Abduction	Knee Extension	Standing heel raise
Movement	Lumbar extension (thorax backward movement away from pelvis)	Lumbar lateral flexion (thorax sideways movement toward pelvis)*	Hip joint extension (upper leg movement straight back)	Hip joint abduction (upper leg movement away from midline to side)	Knee Joint Extension (lower leg movement from bent to straightened position)	Ankle joint extension (plantar flexion) (foot movement by raising heel)
Muscle Most Involved	Erector spinae	Quadratus lumborum	Gluteus maximus	Gluteus medius	Quadriceps	Gastrocnemius
Equipment	L A-C back extension machine	Roman chair	L A-C hip extension machine	L A-C hip abduction machine	L A-C knee extension machine	P-L standing calf machine
Joint	Trunk	Trunk	Hip joint	Hip joint	Knee joint	Ankle joint
Exercise	Abdominal curl	Seated twist	Hanging knee raise	Hip adduction	Prone knee curl	Toe Raise
Movement	Lumbar flexion (thorax forward movement toward pelvis)	Lumbar rotation (thorax twisting movement to one side)	Hip joint flexion (upper leg movement straight forward and upward)	Hip joint adduction (upper leg movement toward midline from side)	Knee joint flexion (lower leg movement from straightened to bent position)	Ankle joint flexion (dorsi flexion) (foot movement by pointing toes upward)
Muscle Most Involved	Rectus abdominis	Obliques	Iliopsoas	Adductor magnus	Hamstrings	Tibialis anterior
Equipment	P-L abdominal machine	L A-C lumbar rotation machine	Captain's chair	L A-C hip adduction machine	L A-C prone knee curl machine	P-L tibialis machine

*Unlike the other paired movements in this table, lumbar lateral flexion and lumbar rotation aren't movements produced by agonist/antagonist muscle groups; they're simply two additional spinal-column movements.

Key: L A-C = lever-arm-and-cam; P-L = plate-loaded

Addenda
to the Day Two
Lower-Body Routine

Cervical extension, flexion, and lateral flexion exercises can be included here in a lower-body routine along with the other spinal-column exercises, as part of a comprehensive spinal workout. Or the cervical exercises can be included in an upper-body routine along with exercises for the shoulder joint because the neck is located near the shoulders, chest, and upper back.

Sets for the cervical spine using a plate-loaded neck machine would comprise the exercises in the table below.

There's another exercise for ankle joint extension (plantar flexion): the seated heel raise. It, too, should be performed as part of your lower-body routine, because it emphasizes a different muscle than the standing heel raise does. Whereas the standing heel raise emphasizes the gastrocnemius, the seated heel raise emphasizes the soleus muscle. This exercise is performed on the plate-loaded seated calf machine.

Upper-Body Routine Featuring Lever-Arm-and-Cam Machines

Pair One: Shoulder Joint

Pec deck fly: shoulder joint horizontal adduction (lever-arm-and-cam pec deck machine)
Reverse pec deck fly: shoulder joint horizontal abduction (lever-arm-and-cam pec deck machine)

Pair Two: Shoulder Joint

Chest press: shoulder joint horizontal adduction (lever-arm-and-cam chest press machine)
High Row: Shoulder joint horizontal abduction (lever-arm-and-cam row machine)

Pair Three: Shoulder Joint

Side raise: shoulder joint abduction (lever-arm-and-cam lateral raise machine)
Lat pulldown: shoulder joint adduction (lever-arm-and-cam lat pulldown machine)

Pair Four: Elbow Joint

Biceps curl: elbow joint flexion (lever-arm-and-cam biceps machine)
Triceps extension: elbow joint extension (lever-arm-and-cam triceps machine)

Cervical Spine Exercises
Using a Plate-Loaded Neck Machine

Exercise	Backward neck bend	Forward neck bend	Sideways neck bend
Movement	Cervical extension (backward movement of the head away from the chest)	Cervical flexion (forward movement of the head toward the chest)	Cervical lateral flexion (sideways movement of the head toward the shoulder)
Muscle most involved	Erector spinae (upper fibers)	Sternocleidomastoid (both sides)	Sternocleidomastoid (left or right)

Pair Five: Shoulder Girdle

Shoulder shrug: shoulder girdle elevation (plate-loaded shrug machine)

Shoulder pulldown: shoulder girdle depression (cable-and-pulley lat pulldown machine)

Pair Six: Shoulder Girdle

Shoulder diagonal raise: shoulder girdle abduction (dumbbell)

Shoulder diagonal pulldown: shoulder girdle adduction (dual cable-and-swivel pulley machine)

DAY FOUR

Lower-Body Routine Featuring Cable-and-Pulley Machines, Plate-Loaded Machines, and Calisthenics Equipment

Pair One: Trunk

Back extension: lumbar extension (Roman chair)

Abdominal curl: lumbar flexion (decline abdominal bench)

Pair Two: Trunk

Side bend: lumbar lateral flexion (Roman chair)

Oblique crunch: lumbar rotation (decline abdominal bench)

Pair Three: Hip Joint

Bent-leg hip extension: hip extension (cable crossover machine)

Sit up: hip flexion (decline abdominal bench)

Pair Four: Hip Joint

Hip abduction: hip joint abduction (cable crossover machine)

Hip adduction: hip joint adduction (cable crossover machine)

Pair Five: Knee Joint

Leg press: knee joint extension (plate-loaded machine)

Lying knee curl: knee joint flexion (cable crossover machine)

Pair Six: Ankle Joint

Standing heel raise: ankle joint extension (plantar flexion) (plate-loaded standing calf machine)

Weighted toe raise: ankle joint flexion (dorsi flexion) (dumbbell)

DAY FIVE

Upper-Body Routine Featuring Free Weights

This upper-body routine may be performed on day five of the weekly routine, or if you prefer performing only four daily routines per week, may be rotated with the two other upper-body routines over three weeks.

Pair One: Shoulder Joint

Flat bench press: shoulder joint horizontal adduction (barbell)

Prone reverse fly: shoulder joint horizontal abduction (dumbbells)

Pair Two: Shoulder Joint

Incline bench press: shoulder joint horizontal adduction (barbell)

Shoulder joint horizontal abduction: t-bar row (plate-loaded machine)

Pair Three: Shoulder Joint

Shoulder press: shoulder joint abduction (dumbbells)

Lat pulldown: shoulder joint adduction (cable-and-pulley lat pulldown machine)

Pair Four: Shoulder Joint

0-to-90-degree front raise: shoulder joint flexion (dumbbells)

0-to-90-degree straight arm pulldown: shoulder joint extension (cable-and-pulley crossover machine)

Pair Five: Shoulder Joint

90-to-180-degree front raise: shoulder joint flexion (dumbbells)

90-to-180-degree straight arm pulldown: shoulder joint extension (cable-and-pulley crossover machine)

Pair Six: Elbow Joint

Standing biceps curl: elbow joint flexion (dumbbells)

French press: elbow joint extension (dumbbell)

Practicing a weekly routine of haphazardly selected exercises is ineffective and inefficient. By putting in place a weekly routine composed of varied yet related daily routines—that is, by putting daily routines in accord with each other over a week—we not only make our weekly routine effective and efficient, we establish a harmonious rhythm to our lives.

A Six-Month Program

The first six months of weight-resistance yoga practice constitutes a strength-training development period.

Progression of Exercises

For the first six months of practice, the novice weight-resistance yogin seeks not only to learn correct technique but also to increase muscular strength. This is accomplished by steadily applying more bodily exertion than usual in obedience to the principle of progressive overload: muscles only become stronger when exercise resistance is gradually increased. The amount of increase in strength is proportional to the amount of increase of overload.

Instruction

If you are an average, healthy adult without training (or without recent training), perform 12 to 15 repetitions of an exercise at a moderate weight, say 60 percent of your maximum capacity, with a restricted range of motion.

When you are able to perform the exercise for one to two repetitions over the targeted number, increase the weight load by 2 to 10 percent, decrease the repetitions, and slightly increase the range of motion.

In this manner, gradually progress until you've reduced the repetitions to a range of 8 to 12 repetitions, increased the weight load to 80 to 85 percent of maximum capacity, and become able to move through the full range of motion. Those of you with recent training may begin with these advanced guidelines.

Once you're able to perform an exercise at 80 to 85 percent of your maximum resistance for 8 to 12 repetitions while reaching temporary failure in under 90 seconds, you may want to advance further. You can progress by increasing the training intensity. There are several ways to do this. One way is to fatigue more fibers.

Instruction

After you've finished a set, continue the set with a reduced resistance. For example, when you can no long press 100 pounds, drop the weight to 80 pounds, and complete two or three additional repetitions. By extending the set in this way, you experience muscle failure twice.

A second way to progress is to have a partner assist with a few additional repetitions at the point of muscle failure.

Instruction

Have your partner provide just enough assistance to enable you to complete the concentric movement (often, a lifting movement), but you perform the eccentric movement (often, a lowering movement) on your own. Two or three assisted negative repetitions performed in this manner (with you resisting the elongation of a muscle group) enable you to fatigue more muscle fibers.

A third way to progress is to vary the repetition/resistance relationship. It's sometimes advantageous to complete more repetitions at a lower resistance or perform fewer repetitions at a higher resistance.

Instruction

Your quadriceps, or pectoralis major, or some other muscle may be so accustomed to performing 10 repetitions at 100 pounds that you should perform 12 repetitions at 90 pounds or 8 repetitions at 110 pounds. Making changes in the repetitions/resistance relationship by having light, moderate, and heavy training days changes muscle fiber recruitment patterns, producing increases in strength.

Due to the greater demands on muscles and the consequent longer period needed for tissue-building, increasing the training intensity by these and other means should be limited to one upper-body and one lower-body exercise routine per week.

During the six-month strength-training development period, weight-resistance yogins become stronger (those who were sedentary become considerably stronger). In contrast to most weight-training systems, which emphasize using various means of continually progressing to higher levels of strength or size, after six months the weight-resistance yoga system becomes a maintenance program that can be continued more or less for the rest of our lives. While some may wish to progress more, most of us are satisfied with maintaining the level we've achieved and unconcerned with eliciting greater strength gains. We accept our limitations. We're grateful for what we can accomplish.

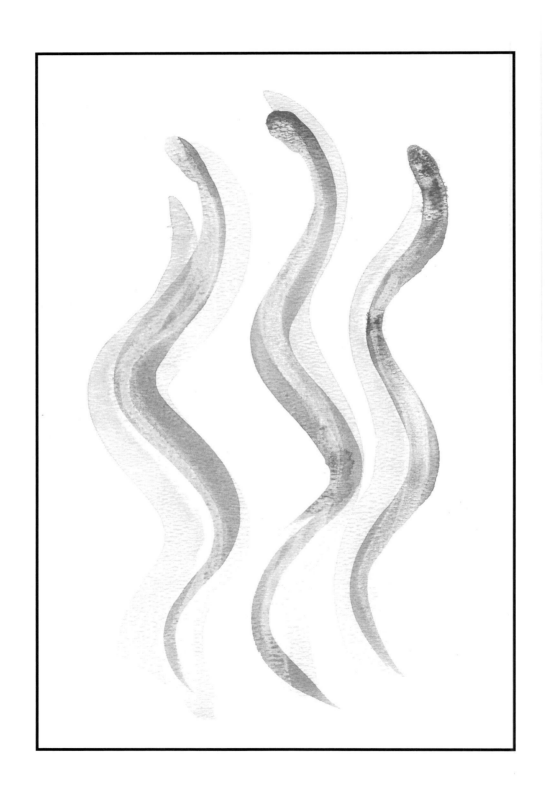

PART TWO

. . . .

Exercise Instructions

Our skeleton is simply incapable of generating movement or supporting itself against gravity without the actions of muscles. Muscles make joints mobile by moving bony levers around a joint axis, and they make joints stable by keeping joint surfaces close and resistant to extraneous movement.

In consideration of these critical muscle functions, weight-resistance yoga sets as its goal not building muscles per se but building muscles in order to systematically enhance joint strength, flexibility, and stability. For this reason, the weight-resistance yoga regimen is organized around exercises for all the major joint movements.

7

EXERCISES FOR THE SHOULDER JOINT

The shoulder joint is formed by the head of the upper arm bone (humerus) loosely fitting into the shallow cavity of the shoulder blade (scapula). This instability allows for great arm mobility.

Muscles from near and far—the deltoid, rotator cuff, and other muscles that originate on the shoulder; the pectoralis major, which originates on the chest; and the latissimus dorsi, infraspinatus, and other muscles that originate on the back—cross the shoulder joint to insert on the upper arm.

The shoulder joint is a ball-and-socket joint, which permits these muscles to produce horizontal, side-to-side, and front-to-back movements of the upper arm:

- turning the arm toward the midline (70° to 90° of internal rotation), an action primarily of the latissimus dorsi, and turning the arm away from the midline (70° to 90° of external rotation), an action primarily of the infraspinatus;
- lowering the arm sideways from the side of the head to across the body (230° to 320° of adduction), an action primarily of the latissimus dorsi, and raising the arm sideways from the side of the body to the side of the head (180° of abduction), an action primarily of the deltoids;
- with the elbows out to the side, moving the arm horizontally toward the chest from the side (135 degrees of horizontal adduction), an action primarily of the pectoralis major, and, with the elbows out to the side, moving the arm horizontally from the front of the chest to behind the back (180° degrees of horizontal abduction), an action primarily of the infraspinatus;
- and raising the arm straight ahead and up from the side of the body (180° degrees of flexion), an action primarily of the anterior deltoid and upper pectoralis major, and lowering the arm from the side of the head to behind the body (225° to 240° degrees of extension), an action primarily of the posterior deltoid and latissimus dorsi.

These upper arm movements performed against resistance strengthen the shoulder joint muscles to make everyday lifting and lowering and pushing and pulling activities (such as pushing a cart and hauling out the trash) easier.

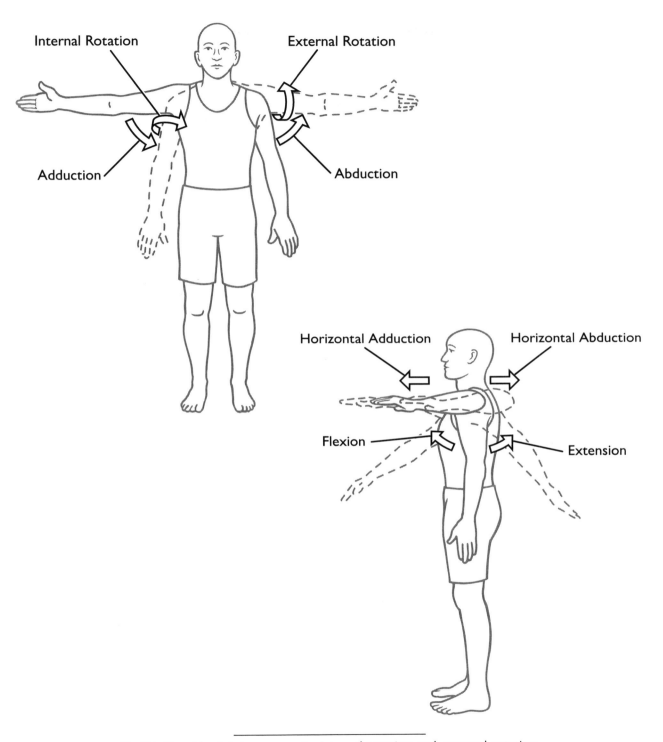

Fig. 7.1. Shoulder joint movements: internal rotation and external rotation, adduction and abduction, horizontal adduction and horizontal abduction, and flexion and extension

Lat Pulldown
Cable Lat Pulldown Machine

Joint movements: shoulder joint adduction and extension

Shoulder joint adduction is downward movement of the upper arm from the side toward the midline of the body. Shoulder joint extension is movement of the upper arm straight backward.

Muscles most involved in joint movements: latissimus dorsi, teres major, and lower pectoralis major

POSITIONING

1. Grab the bar with a wide, palm-facing-away grip, and sit down with your thighs and lower legs at a right angle and your feet, slightly pigeon-toed, firmly on the floor.
2. Bend your elbows until your upper arms are at 90° from your side (at shoulder height).
3. Lean slightly back, crisply bring your shoulders down, squeeze your shoulder blades together, and keep your chest up.

MOVEMENT

1. Bring your arms down and slightly back (in slight extension), and rotate your shoulder blades down until the bar reaches your collarbone.
2. Return to the starting position.

COMMON ERRORS	CORRECTIONS
During Muscle-Shortening Phase	
In Movement	
▪ Yanking the bar down.	▪ Pulling the bar down with control.
In Stillness	
▪ Arching the lower back and letting the head go back.	▪ Maintaining the natural curves of the spine by co-tightening the abdomen and lower back.
	▪ Keeping the head and back aligned
During Muscle-Lengthening Phase	
In Movement	
▪ Letting the arms fly up.	▪ Restricting arm movement to 90° (at shoulder height).
▪ Stopping at the top to "load up."	▪ Moving continuously (to maintain tension).
In Stillness	
▪ Scrunching up the shoulders.	▪ Keeping the shoulders down.
▪ Lifting off the seat.	▪ Sitting firmly on the seat.

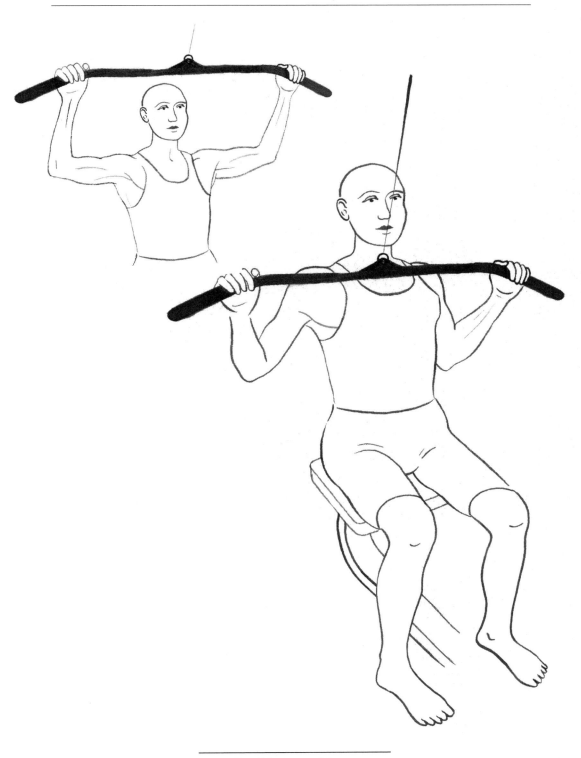

Fig. 7.2. Lat pulldown

45-to-90-Degree Shoulder Press

Dumbbells

Joint movements: shoulder joint abduction
Shoulder joint abduction is upward movement of the upper arm out to the side, away from the midline of the body.

Muscles most involved in joint movements: latissimus dorsi, teres major, and lower pectoralis major

POSITIONING

1. Pick up the dumbbells, and sit on a seat with an inclined back. (No other exercise creates so much pressure on the lower back as the overhead press; a seat with an inclined back alleviates the compression.)
2. Thrust the dumbbells up to your shoulders (with the inner plates resting on the tips of your shoulders).
3. Spread your legs shoulder-width apart.
4. Slightly lift the dumbbells from your shoulders. Your forearms should be at a diagonal to the floor, and your elbows should be pointed out to the sides.

MOVEMENT

1. Powerfully contract your abdominals to firmly hold your spine in place.
2. Move your arms up until your upper arms are approximately parallel to the floor (between 90° and 110°) and your forearms are perpendicular to the floor.
3. Return to the starting position.

COMMON ERRORS	CORRECTIONS
During Muscle-Shortening Phase	
In Movement	
■ Flinging up the dumbbells.	■ Raising the dumbbells slowly.
In Stillness	
■ Scrunching up the shoulders.	■ Keeping the shoulders down.
■ Arching the back to gain leverage (mechanical advantage) to produce momentum for lifting the weight.	■ Keeping the trunk stable and erect by co-tightening the abdomen and lower back.
During Muscle-Lengthening Phase	
In Movement	
■ Lowering the dumbbells too quickly.	■ Maintaining vigilance on the lowering movement when great pressure is being placed on the spine (if there's lower back pain, reduce the weight).

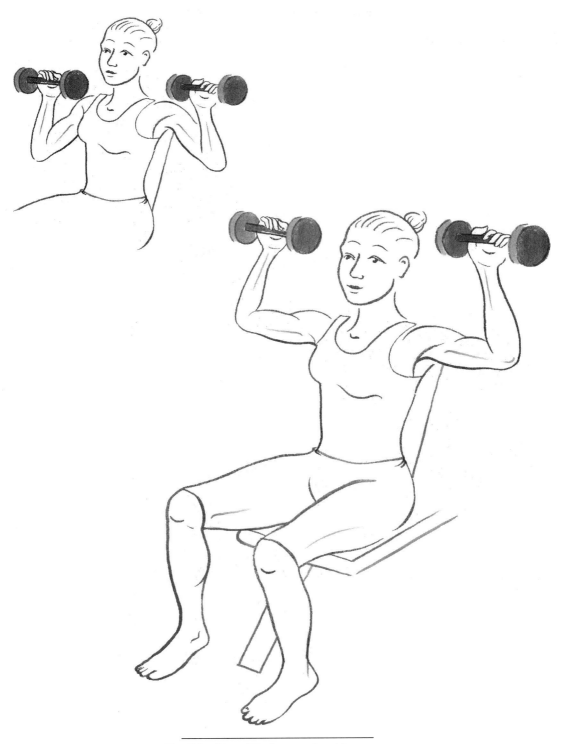

Fig. 7.3. 45-to-90-degree shoulder press

Seated Low Row

Cable Rowing Machine

Joint movements: shoulder joint extension
Shoulder joint extension is movement of the upper arm straight backward.

Muscles most involved in joint movements: latissimus dorsi, teres major, and lower pectoralis major

POSITIONING

1. Sit on the seat, and lean forward to grab a double D handle with a neutral grip.
2. Sit back with your knees slightly bent. Rotate your pelvis back so you're resting squarely on your sitting bones.
3. Slightly bend your stretched-out arms at the elbows. Squeeze your shoulder blades together, and keep your chest up. Maintain the natural curves of your back.

MOVEMENT

1. Move your upper arms from in front of your chest down, out, and back until your elbows are at least 30° to the side (to increase the angle of pull of the lats) and behind your trunk, and simultaneously move your shoulder blades yet closer to the spine (and one another).
2. Return to the starting position.

COMMON ERRORS	CORRECTIONS
During Muscle-Shortening Phase	
In Movement	
▪ Yanking the arms back.	▪ Pulling the handle back slowly and with control.
In Stillness	
▪ Arching the lower back to help jerk the weight back.	▪ Keeping the natural curves of the spine by co-tightening the abdomen and lower back.
▪ Straightening the legs.	▪ Keeping the legs slightly bent.
▪ Raising the shoulders.	▪ Keeping the shoulders down.
During Muscle-Lengthening Phase	
In Movement	
▪ Letting the arms go slack.	▪ Maintaining tension in the arms.
In Stillness	
▪ Letting the shoulder blades go slack.	▪ Resisting the inevitable movement of the shoulder blades away from the spinal column.
▪ Letting the trunk be pulled forward.	▪ Keeping the trunk erect.

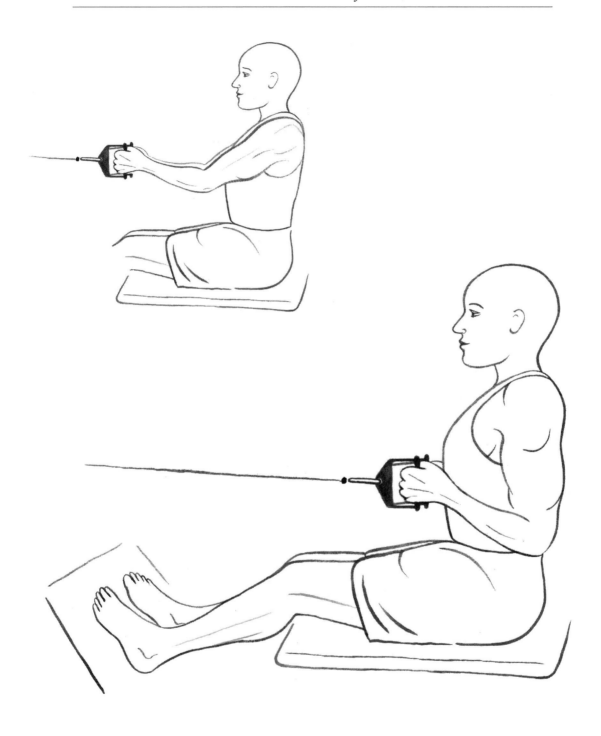

Fig. 7.4. Seated low row

0-to-90-Degree Front Raise

Dumbbells

Joint movements: shoulder joint flexion and internal rotation
Shoulder joint flexion is movement of the upper arm straight forward. Shoulder joint internal rotation is the movement of the upper arm around its long axis toward the midline.

Muscles most involved in joint movements: anterior deltoid and upper pectoralis major

POSITIONING
1. Stand holding dumbbells with a palms-facing-up grip at the front of your thighs.
2. Spread your legs shoulder-width apart to achieve stability. If more stability is needed, slightly bend your knees, while remaining erect.
3. Pinch your shoulder blades together.
4. Slightly raise your arms.

MOVEMENT
1. Lift an arm directly forward while inwardly rotating it. Bring the outstretched arm up to shoulder height (no more, no less).
2. Return to the starting position.
3. Alternate the action with the other arm.

COMMON ERRORS	CORRECTIONS
During Muscle-Shortening Phase	
In Movement	
▪ Lifting the dumbbells above or below the shoulder.	▪ Lifting the dumbbells to shoulder height.
▪ Using momentum.	▪ Lifting the dumbbells moderately slowly (you should be able to stop the upward movement at any position in its arc).
▪ Bending the elbows (in order to handle too heavy weights).	▪ Keeping the elbows straight (or slightly bent if discomfort is felt).
In Stillness	
▪ Scrunching up the shoulders.	▪ Keeping the shoulders down.
▪ Arching the back to gain leverage (mechanical advantage) for flinging up the dumbbells.	▪ Keeping the trunk stable by co-tightening the abdomen and lower back.
During Muscle-Lengthening Phase	
In Movement	
▪ Lowering the dumbbells too quickly.	▪ Lowering the dumbbells moderately slowly (you should be able to stop the downward movement at any position in its arc).

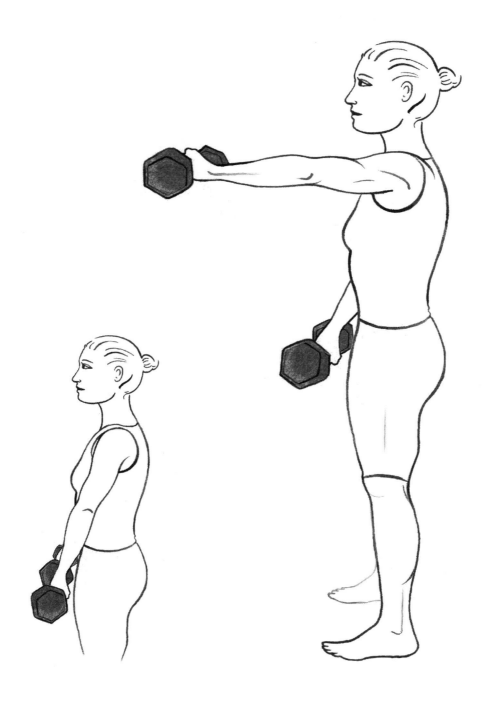

Fig. 7.5. 0-to-90-degree front raise

Standing High Row

Dual Cable and Swivel Pulley Machine

Joint movements: shoulder joint horizontal abduction and external rotation
Shoulder joint horizontal abduction is horizontal movement of the upper arm away from the chest. Shoulder joint external rotation is movement of the upper arm around its long axis away from the midline.

Muscles most involved in joint movements: rear deltoids, teres minor, and infraspinatus

POSITIONING

1. Stand facing away from the machine. Cross your arms, and grab the handles with a palm-facing-down grip.
2. Move your elbows out until they're shoulder-width apart (left hand over right elbow, and right hand below left elbow). Your arms should be horizontal to the floor and crossed in front of your chest just below the tops of your shoulders.
3. Squeeze your shoulder blades together.

MOVEMENT

1. Keeping your elbows high without raising your shoulders, move your upper arms back until they're extended straight out to the sides, and simultaneously externally rotate your upper arms until your forearms are vertical.
2. Return to the starting position.

COMMON ERRORS	CORRECTIONS
During Muscle-Shortening Phase	
In Movement	
▪ Limiting the full range of motion by not pulling the elbows beyond the plane of the back and not making the forearms upright.	▪ Fully bringing back and outwardly rotating the upper arms (elbows parallel to trunk, forearms vertical, and upper arms horizontal).
▪ Lowering the elbows.	
In Stillness	
▪ Raising the shoulders.	▪ Keeping the shoulders down.
▪ Lurching with the lower back.	▪ Keeping the trunk stable by co-contracting the muscles of the abdomen and lower back.
During Muscle-Lengthening Phase	
In Movement	
▪ Letting the arms go slack.	▪ Maintaining tension in the arms by keeping them slightly bent.
In Stillness	
▪ Quickly releasing the shoulder blades.	▪ Releasing the shoulder blades and arms slowly.
▪ Letting the chest be pulled forward.	▪ Keeping the chest up.

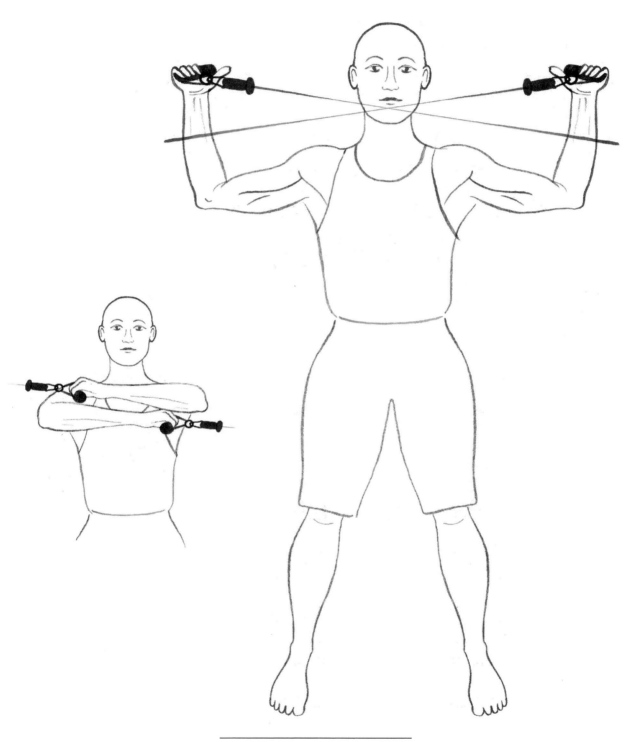

Fig. 7.6. Standing high row

Flat Bench Press

Barbell

Joint movements: shoulder joint horizontal adduction
Shoulder joint horizontal adduction is horizontal movement of the upper arm toward and across the chest.

Muscles most involved in joint movements: pectoralis major, anterior deltoid, and coracobrachialis

POSITIONING

1. Lie on your back on the bench. Plant your feet flat on the floor, shoulder width apart. Grab the bar at slightly wider than shoulder width.
2. Unrack the bar from the stands. Retract your shoulder blades (to provide the stability that allows for the pressing movement), flair your "wings" (static lats help stabilize the trunk and guide the pressing movement), and slightly tuck in your elbows (to protect your shoulders).
3. Lower the bar close to your chest.

MOVEMENT

1. Straighten your arms to lift the bar up in a straight line, and simultaneously drive your shoulders into the bench.
2. Return to the starting position.
3. Rack the bar at the top of the last repetition (after the last concentric contraction).

COMMON ERRORS	CORRECTIONS
During Muscle-Shortening Phase	
In Movement	
▪ Locking the elbows.	▪ Keeping the elbows slightly bent.
▪ Pushing the bar back (over the face).	▪ Keeping the bar straight up (away from the face).
In Stillness	
▪ Relaxing the shoulder blades.	▪ Driving the shoulders and middle of the back into the bench to resist the inevitable forward movement of the shoulder blades.
▪ Arching the back and thrusting the glutes off the bench.	▪ Keeping the lower back in its natural arch by co-tightening the abdomen and lower back and keeping the pelvis down.
During Muscle-Lengthening Phase	
In Movement	
▪ Stopping the downward motion before the "sticking point" is reached.	▪ Lowering the bar close to the chest.
▪ Bouncing the bar off the chest.	

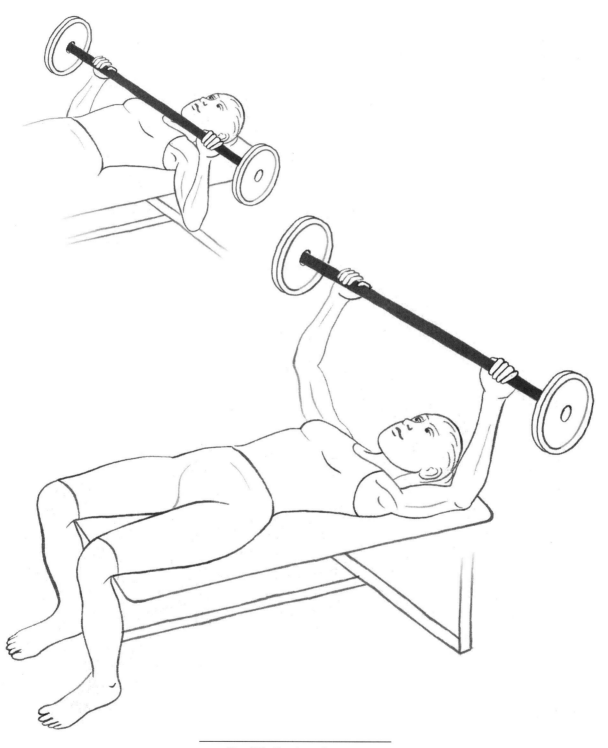

Fig. 7.7. Flat bench press

8

EXERCISES FOR
THE ELBOW JOINT

The elbow joint is actually composed of two interrelated joints. One joint is formed by a part of the upper arm (humerus) securely fitting into the notch of the larger forearm bone (ulna) at the humeroulnar joint. The other joint is formed by a nearby part of the upper arm (humerus) having weak contact with the smaller forearm bone (radius) at the radiohumeral joint.

The biceps (biceps brachii, brachialis, and brachioradialis), which originate on the front shoulder and upper arm, cross both of these joints to insert on the front of the forearm; and the triceps, which originate on the back shoulder and upper arm, cross the just the humeroulnar joint to insert on the back of the forearm.

The less critical radioulnar joint is a pivot joint, which permits its muscles to produce only rotational movements of the forearm:

- with the hand facing forward, twisting the forearm inward so the palm faces back (70° to 90° of internal rotation, or pronation), an action of the brachioradialis, and, with the hand facing backward, twisting the forearm outward so the palm faces forward (70° to 90° of external rotation, or supination), an action of the biceps brachii and brachioradialis.

The humeroulnar joint—the primary site of elbow joint motion—is a hinge joint, which permits its muscles to produce only front-to-back movements of the forearm:

- bending the forearm from the straightened position (145° to 150° of flexion), an action of the biceps, and straightening the forearm from the bent position (145° to 150° of extension), an action of the triceps.

These lower arm movements performed against resistance strengthen the muscles of the elbow joint to make everyday forearm activities (such as pulling open a door and twisting a screwdriver) easier.

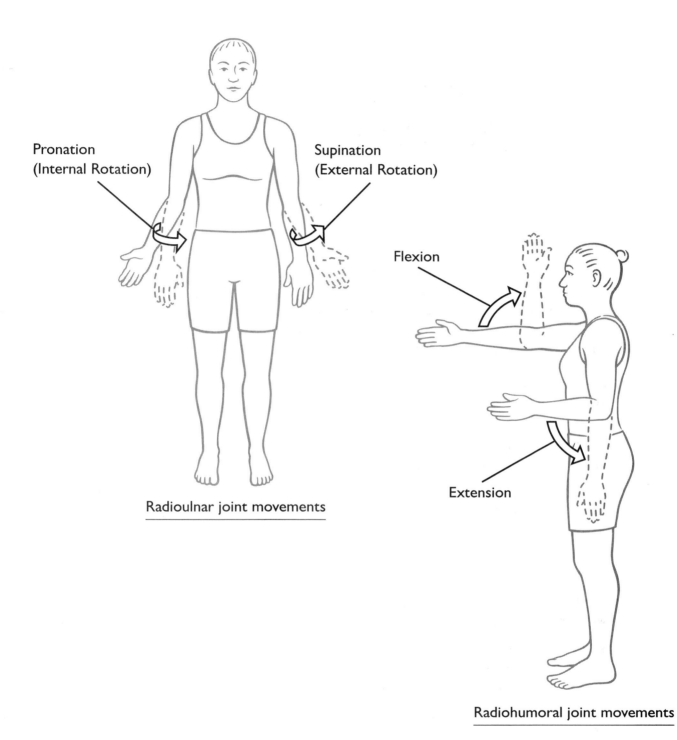

Pronation
(Internal Rotation)

Supination
(External Rotation)

Radioulnar joint movements

Flexion

Extension

Radiohumoral joint movements

Fig. 8.1. Elbow joint movements: pronation and supination
and flexion and extension

Standing Biceps Curl

Dumbbells

Joint movements: elbow joint flexion and supination
Elbow joint flexion is the movement of the forearm toward the shoulder by bending the elbow, thereby decreasing the angle between the shoulder and the forearm. Supination is the external rotary movement of the forearm that results in the hand moving from the palm-down to the palm-up position.

Muscles most involved in joint movements: biceps brachii, brachialis, and brachioradialis

POSITIONING

1. Stand with your feet slightly wider than shoulder-width apart. Hold the dumbbells at your front thighs with a palms-facing-down grip.
2. Lightly touch your elbows to your sides. Bend your elbows just enough to allow your forearms to slightly lift the dumbbells away from your thighs.

MOVEMENT

1. While keeping your upper arms fixed, bend and outwardly rotate your forearms until your palms face inward again as you lift the dumbbells to chest height.
2. Return to the starting position.

COMMON ERRORS	CORRECTIONS
During Muscle-Shortening Phase	
In Movement	
■ Shifting the elbows back and then swinging the forearms up to gain momentum.	■ Keeping the elbows at the sides.
■ Raising the dumbbells to a nearly 180° angle, at the chest.	■ Raising the dumbbells to only a 135° angle, to maintain tension (tension is greatest at 90°, when the forearms are parallel to the floor, and steadily decreases thereafter).
In Stillness	
■ Tilting the head back.	■ Keeping the head erect.
■ Swinging the upper arms up.	■ Keeping the upper arms down and the shoulders back.
■ Pushing the pelvic girdle forward by arching the lower back to gain momentum with a rocking movement.	■ Keeping the torso erect by co-tightening the abdomen and lower back.
During Muscle-Lengthening Phase	
In Movement	
■ Lowering the dumbbells quickly.	■ Lowering the dumbbells with control.

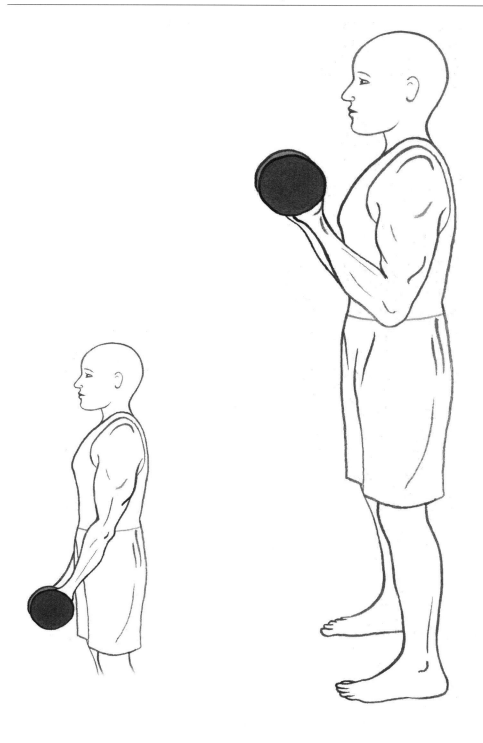

Fig. 8.2. Standing biceps curl

Triceps Pushdown
Cable Triceps Machine

Joint movements: elbow joint extension and pronation
Elbow joint extension is movement of the forearm away from the shoulder by straightening the elbow, thereby increasing the angle between the shoulder and the forearm. Pronation is internal rotary movement of the forearm that results in the hand moving from the palm-up to the palm-down position.

Muscles most involved in joint movements: triceps brachii and brachioradialis

POSITIONING
1. Stand with your feet slightly wider than shoulder-width apart.
2. Hold the handles with a narrow, palms-facing-up grip, and bend your elbows to bring the handles to chest level.
3. Lightly touch your elbows to your sides.

MOVEMENT
1. While keeping your upper arms fixed, push down to straighten your arms while simultaneously inwardly rotating your forearms.
2. Return to the starting position.

COMMON ERRORS	CORRECTIONS
During Muscle-Shortening Phase	
In Movement	
▪ Bringing the elbows back.	▪ Holding the elbows in place (they are the fulcrum).
▪ Letting the elbows drift out to the side.	
In Stillness	
▪ Bending the wrists far back.	▪ Keeping the wrists slightly bent back.
▪ Scrunching up the shoulders.	▪ Keeping the shoulders down.
▪ Bending, hunching, or leaning forward.	▪ Standing up straight.
During Muscle-Lengthening Phase	
In Movement	
▪ Letting the forearms fly up.	▪ Bringing the forearms up slowly and with control.

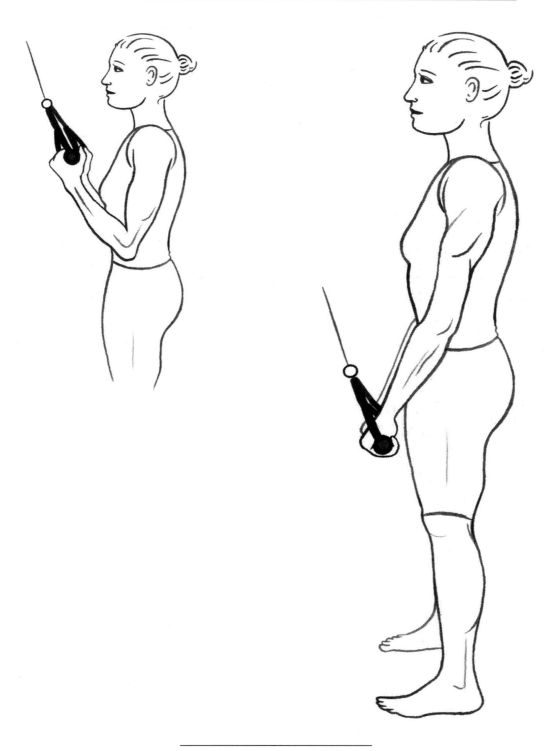

Fig. 8.3. Triceps pushdown

9

EXERCISES FOR THE SHOULDER GIRDLE

The shoulder girdle is composed of the collarbones (clavicles), which connect to the sternum at the sternoclavicular joint, and of the shoulder blades (scapulae), which connect to the collarbones at the acromioclavicular joint. Shoulder girdle joint motion primarily occurs at the sternoclavicular joint—the only location where the shoulder girdle (and, by extension, the arms) connects to the main skeleton. Movement of the shoulder blades on the spine and rib cage, however, is defined by the scapulothoracic joint, which isn't a true joint because its movements are totally dependent on the sternoclavicular and acromioclavicular joints.

The trapezius, levator scapulae, and rhomboids, which principally originate on the shoulder blades, insert on the spinal column, and the serratus anterior and pectoralis minor, which originate on the ribs, insert on the shoulder blades.

The scapulothoracic joint permits these muscles to produce movements of the shoulder blades:

- shrugging the shoulders from the resting position (50° of elevation), an action of the rhomboids and upper and middle trapezius, and lowering the shoulders from near the ears (55° degrees of depression), an action of the lower trapezius and pectoralis minor;
- swiveling the shoulder blades up (30° of upward rotation), an action of the trapezius and lower serratus anterior, and swiveling the shoulder blades down from the rotated up position (30° of downward rotation), action of the rhomboids and pectoralis minor;
- and splaying the shoulder blades from the resting position (15 degrees of abduction, or protraction), an action of the upper serratus anterior and pectoralis minor, and squeezing the shoulder blades together from the spread forward position (35° of adduction, or retraction), an action of the middle trapezius and rhomboids.

These shoulder blade movements performed against resistance strengthen the shoulder girdle muscles to provide a fixed yet yielding point from which the arms can exert force, thus contributing to everyday arm activities (such as pushing the arms down to get up from a chair or raising the arms to put a book on a shelf).

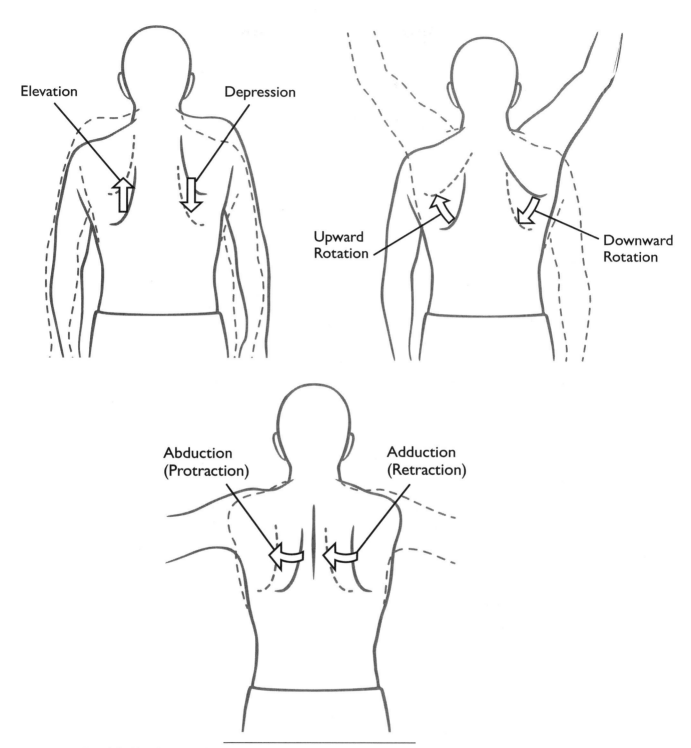

Fig. 9.1. Shoulder girdle movements: elevation and depression, upward rotation and downward rotation, and abduction and adduction

Shoulder Pulldown

Cable Lat Pulldown Machine

Joint movements: shoulder girdle depression, downward rotation, and adduction (retraction)

Shoulder girdle depression is downward movement of the shoulder blade to the resting position. Shoulder girdle downward rotation is movement of the bottom tip of the shoulder blade inward and toward the spinal column to the resting position. Shoulder girdle adduction (retraction) is movement of the shoulder blade backward toward the spinal column.

Muscles most involved in joint movements: lower trapezius and rhomboids

POSITIONING

1. Reach up to grab the bar with a wide grip. Sit squarely on your sitz bones with your trunk erect, while straightening your elbows.
2. Keeping your shoulders up around your ears, slightly lower your shoulders.

MOVEMENT

1. While keeping your arms straight, pull your shoulders down, and simultaneously rotate your shoulder blades downward toward your spine and bring your shoulder blades back toward your spine.
2. Return to the starting position.

COMMON ERRORS	CORRECTIONS
During Muscle-Shortening Phase	
In Movement	
■ Bending the elbows to initiate the shoulder movement with the arms.	■ Keeping the elbows straight, allowing the shoulders to lower without the aid of the arms.
In Stillness	
■ Tilting backward.	■ Maintaining erect posture.
During Muscle-Lengthening Phase	
In Movement	
■ Quickly releasing the shoulders (letting them fly up).	■ Releasing the shoulders under tension.
In Stillness	
■ Tilting forward.	■ Maintaining erect posture.

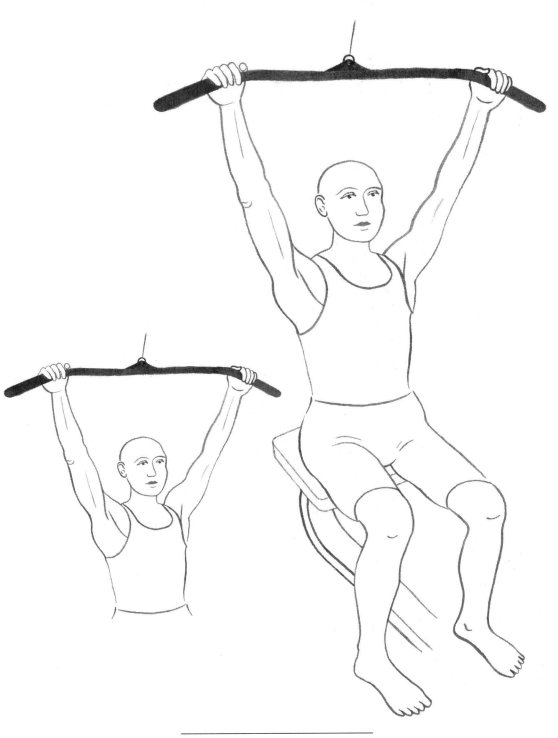

Fig. 9.2. Shoulder pulldown

Shoulder Shrug

Plate-Loaded Shrug Machine

Joint movements: shoulder girdle elevation, upward rotation, and adduction (retraction) Shoulder girdle elevation is upward movement of the shoulder blade. Shoulder girdle upward rotation is movement of the bottom tip of the shoulder blade outward and away from the spinal column. Shoulder girdle adduction (retraction) is movement of the shoulder blade backward toward the spinal column.

Muscles most involved in joint movements: upper and middle trapezius, rhomboids, and levator scapulae

POSITIONING

1. Bend at the knees, and grab the handles at the sides of your body.
2. Stand erect by straightening your knees.
3. Slightly raise your shoulders.

MOVEMENT

1. Lift your shoulders as high as you can, hiding your neck, and simultaneously rotate your shoulder blades up and pull your shoulder blades back toward the spine and each other. Keep your head in place, focusing directly in front of you.
2. Return to the starting position.

COMMON ERRORS	CORRECTIONS
During Muscle-Shortening Phase	
In Movement	
▪ Rounding the shoulders.	▪ Pulling the shoulders back until there's an expansive feeling throughout the chest.
In Stillness	
▪ Dropping the head forward or back.	▪ Keeping the head neutral.
▪ Arching the back.	▪ Keeping the natural curve of the lower spine by co-tightening the abdomen and lower back.
▪ Bending the arms to lift the weight.	▪ Keeping the arms straight.
▪ Using the legs to bend and then thrust the weight up.	▪ Keeping the legs straight.
During Muscle-Lengthening Phase	
In Movement	
▪ Lowering the shoulders by letting them go slack.	▪ Lowering the shoulders slowly, resisting the pull of gravity.

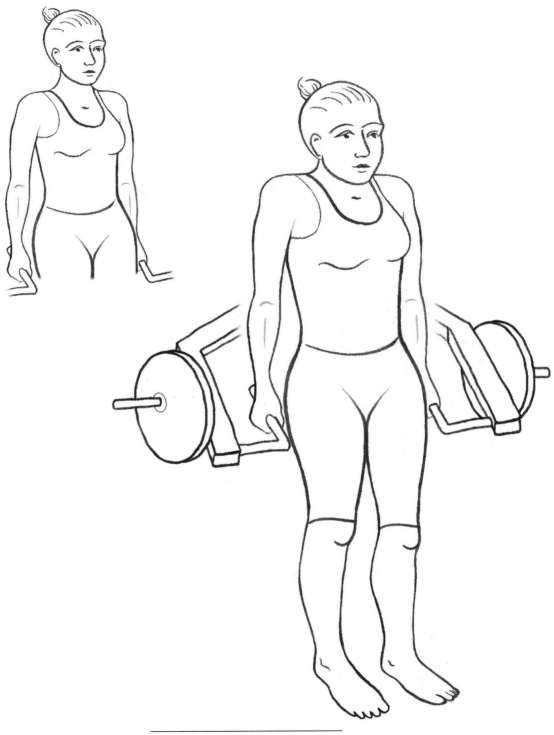

Fig. 9.3. Shoulder shrug

Shoulder Diagonal Pulldown

Dual Cable and Swivel Pulley Machine

Joint movements: shoulder girdle adduction (retraction) and downward rotation
Shoulder girdle adduction (retraction) is movement of the shoulder blade backward toward the spinal column. Shoulder girdle downward rotation is movement of the bottom tip of the shoulder blade inward toward the spinal column to the resting position.

Muscles most involved in joint movements: rhomboids and lower trapezius

POSITIONING

1. While standing, hold the handles, palms facing you, at forehead height in front of your body's midline. With your elbows bent at 90°, make your forearms perpendicular to the floor.
2. Slightly raise the tip of your shoulders.

MOVEMENT

1. Roll your shoulders backward and down while moving your arms diagonally out to the side away from the body's front midline. At the midpoint, your shoulder blades are squeezed together and fully down.
2. Return to the starting position.

COMMON ERRORS	CORRECTIONS
During Muscle-Shortening Phase	
In Movement	
■ Initiating the movement with the arms instead of the shoulder blades.	■ Initiating the movement with the shoulder blades instead of the arms.
■ Rolling the shoulders back to merely a neutral position.	■ Rolling the shoulders completely back (thus fully retracting the shoulders).
■ Keeping the tip of the shoulder up.	■ Pulling the tips of the shoulders fully down (thus fully downwardly rotating the shoulders).
In Stillness	
■ Twisting the torso.	■ Keeping the trunk facing forward by engaging the obliques that oppose the tendency to twist.
■ Changing the 90° angle of the elbows.	■ Maintaining the 90° angle of the elbows.
During Muscle-Lengthening Phase	
In Movement	
■ Returning the elbows to less than the body's midline.	■ Moving the elbows to the body's midline.
■ Scrunching up the shoulders (by recruiting the upper and middle trapezius).	■ Raising only the tips of the shoulders.

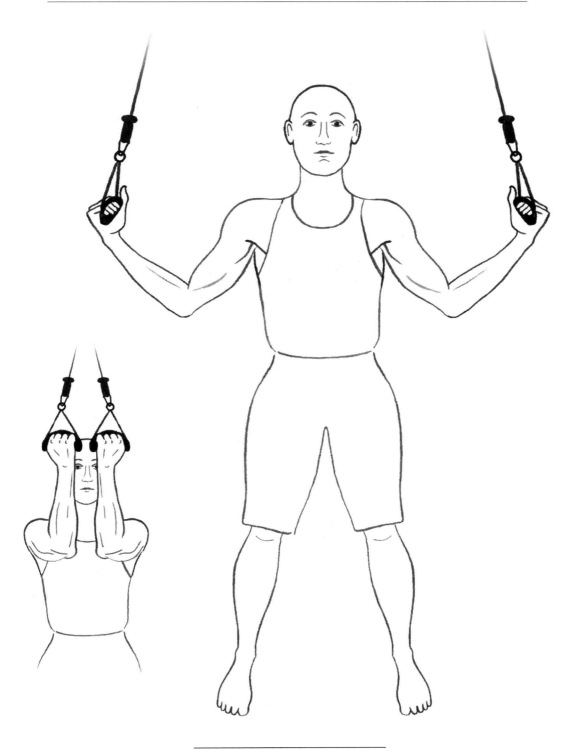

Fig. 9.4. Shoulder diagonal pulldown

Shoulder Diagonal Raise

Dumbbell

Joint movements: shoulder girdle abduction (protraction) and upward rotation
Shoulder girdle abduction (protraction) is movement of the shoulder blade forward and away from the spinal column. Shoulder girdle upward rotation is movement of the bottom tip of the shoulder blade outward and away from the spinal column.

Muscles most involved in joint movements: serratus anterior, pectoralis minor, and middle trapezius

POSITIONING

1. While seated, hold a light dumbbell in one hand. Bend your elbow 90° and out to the side.
2. Roll your shoulder blade back until you feel tightness in your mid-upper back. Keep your shoulder blade down.

MOVEMENT

1. Roll your shoulder forward and up while moving your arm diagonally to the body's front midline. Raise just the tip of your shoulder. At the midpoint, your forearm is perpendicular to the floor, and your hand, palm facing you, is at forehead height.
2. Return to the starting position.
3. After completing the set, repeat the action with the other side.

COMMON ERRORS	CORRECTIONS
During Muscle-Shortening Phase	
In Movement	
▪ Initiating the movement with the arm instead of the shoulder blade.	▪ Initiating the movement with the shoulder blade instead of the arm.
▪ Moving the elbow to less than the body's midline.	▪ Moving the elbow to the body's midline (thus fully protracting the shoulder).
▪ Scrunching up the shoulder (by recruiting the upper and middle trapezius).	▪ Raising the tip of the shoulder (thus fully upwardly rotating the shoulder), not the entire shoulder.
In Stillness	
▪ Twisting the torso.	▪ Keeping the trunk immobile by engaging the obliques to oppose the tendency to twist.
▪ Changing the 90° angle of the elbow.	▪ Maintaining the 90° angle of the elbow.
During Muscle-Lengthening Phase	
In Movement	
▪ Returning the shoulder to the starting position without resisting the pull of gravity.	▪ Returning the shoulder to the starting position while resisting the pull of gravity.

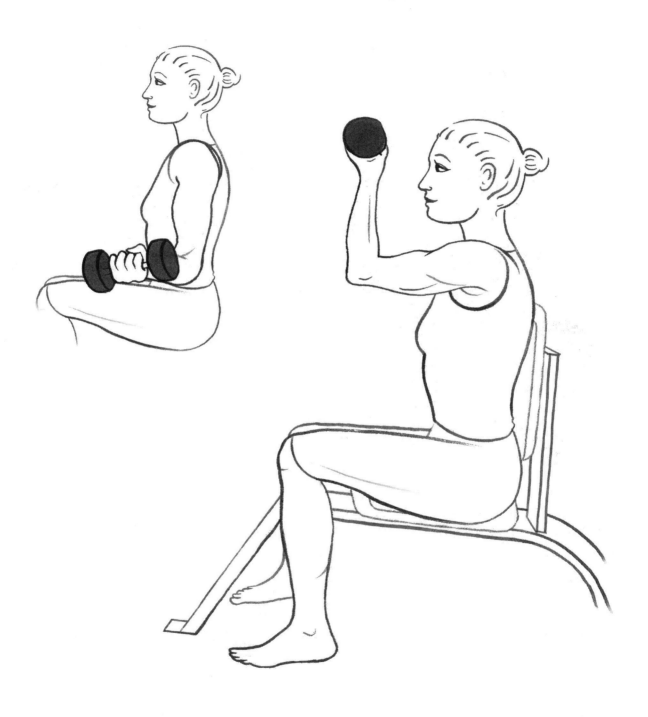

Fig. 9.5. Shoulder diagonal raise

10

EXERCISES FOR THE TRUNK
(VERTEBRAL COLUMN AND ABDOMINAL WALL)

The trunk comprises the spine, or backbone (vertebral column), and the ribs and the breastbone, or sternum. The spine, where the critical trunk joints are located, consists of 24 moving vertebrae: 7 cervical vertebrae; 12 thoracic vertebrae; and 5 lumbar vertebrae (the 5 vertebrae of the sacrum and the 4 vertebrae of the coccyx are fused). The ribs connect with the spine in the back and with the breastbone in the front.

The large muscle of the vertebral column, the erector spinae, originates on the sacrum, lower vertebrae, and ribs and inserts on the upper vertebrae, ribs, and skull. The abdominal wall muscles, the abdominals and quadratus lumborum, either originate on the sternum and ribs and insert on the pelvis or originate on the pelvis and insert on the sternum and ribs.

The major trunk movements occur in the thoracic and lumbar regions of the spine. The two sets of facet joints of the 17 thoracic and lumbar vertebrae are gliding joints, which permit these muscles to produce only limited intervertebral movement. However, although little movement is possible between any two thoracic or lumbar vertebrae, the combined movement of several adjacent vertebrae—especially of the lumbar vertebrae—allows for substantial trunk movement:

- bending the trunk sideways (20° to 40° degrees of lumbar lateral flexion), an action of quadratus lumborum;
- bending the trunk forward from the resting position (70° to 90° of lumbar flexion), an action of the abdominals, and, from the bent forward position, straightening and then bending back the trunk (90° to 120° of lumbar extension), an action of the erector spinae;
- and twisting the trunk (30° to 45° of lumbar rotation), an action of the abdominals.

These trunk movements performed against resistance strengthen the vertebral column and abdominal wall muscles to protect the viscera and the fragile spinal cord; to make everyday lifting and lowering activities that involve the trunk (such as picking up a box from the floor) easier; and to maintain erect posture.

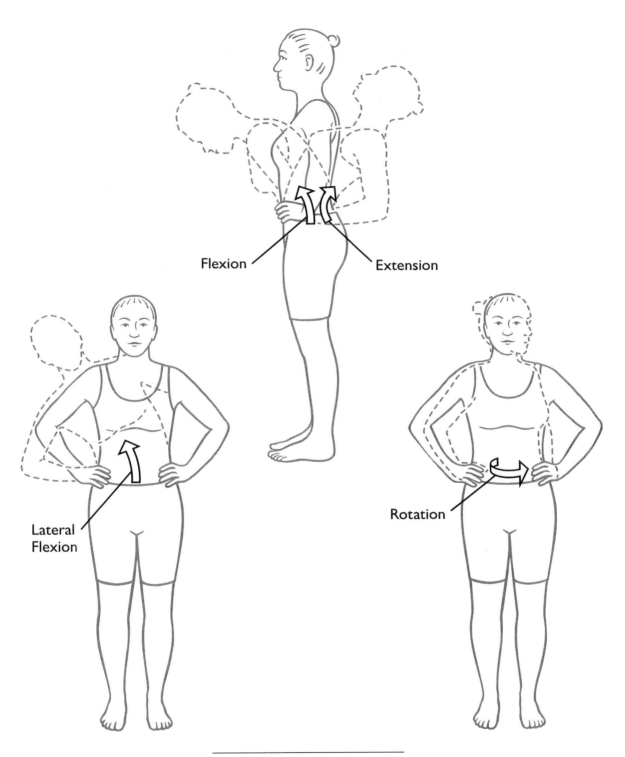

Flexion

Extension

Lateral
Flexion

Rotation

Fig. 10.1. Trunk movements: lumbar lateral flexion, lumbar flexion and extension,
and lumbar rotation

Back Raise

Roman Chair

Joint movements: lumbar extension

Lumbar extension is backward movement of the thorax away from the pelvis.

Muscles most involved in joint movements: erector spinae and multifidus

POSITIONING

1. Lie face down with your entire pelvis resting on the seat (not in front of it).
2. Straighten your legs, and secure your feet on the stand. Point your toes slightly inward.
3. Fold your hands across your chest. Lower your trunk until your back is rounded.
4. Slightly lift your trunk.
   Note: To increase the difficulty, hold a plate at your chest.

MOVEMENT

1. Gradually unfold your back by raising first your upper trunk and then your lower trunk. At the midpoint, your lower back is arched, while your pelvis and thighs remain in the same place as at the beginning.
2. Briefly hold the position, and then return to the starting position.

COMMON ERRORS	CORRECTIONS
During Muscle-Shortening Phase	
In Movement	
▪ Snapping the trunk up.	▪ Raising the back one vertebra at a time.
▪ Keeping the back straight.	▪ Arching the back.
▪ Immediately lowering the back after reaching the midpoint.	▪ Briefly holding the back up at the midpoint to work the deep stabilizing multifidus.
In Stillness	
▪ Tightening the buttocks and back thighs, rotating the pelvis anteriorly, and extending the hips to hyperextend the lower back.	▪ Relaxing the buttocks and back thighs, tilting the pelvis posteriorly, and keeping the hips neutral to prevent hyperextension of the back.
▪ Bending the head back.	▪ Keeping the head aligned with the trunk.
During Muscle-Lengthening Phase	
In Movement	
▪ Keeping the back straight, thereby restricting the range of stretching.	▪ Curling down to achieve a wide range of spinal stretching.
▪ Fully hanging down (which totally relaxes the spinal muscles).	▪ Maintaining tension by stopping short of the full downward range of motion.
In Stillness	
▪ Tucking in the chin	▪ Keeping the head aligned with the trunk.

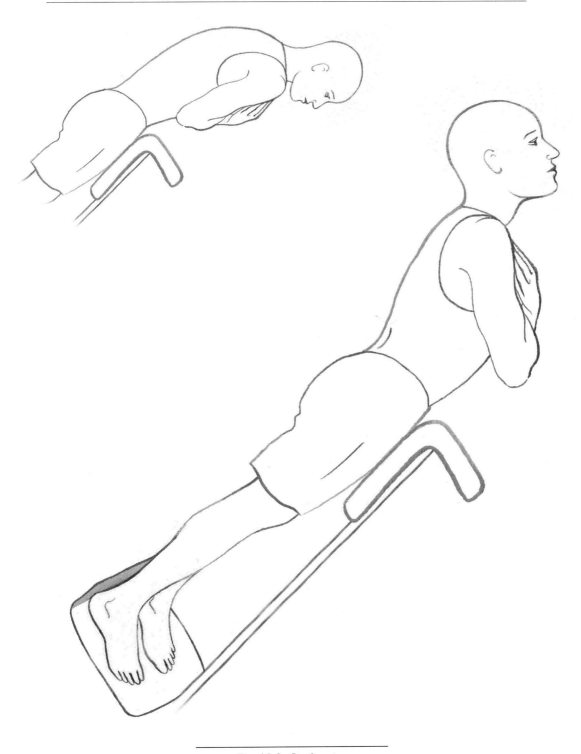

Fig. 10.2. Back raise

Side Bend

Roman Chair

Joint movements: lumbar lateral flexion
Lumbar lateral flexion is the sideways movement of the thorax toward the pelvis.

Muscles most involved in joint movements: quadratus lumborum, rectus abdominis, external oblique, and erector spinae (on one side) and internal oblique (on the opposite side)

POSITIONING

1. Lie sideways with your hips on the seat and your trunk unsupported.
2. Lower your trunk as low as possible.
   Note: To increase the difficulty, clasp a dumbbell or plate to your chest.

MOVEMENT

1. Raise your trunk as high as possible.
2. Briefly hold the position.
3. Return to the starting position.
4. After completing the set, repeat the action with the other side.

COMMON ERRORS	CORRECTIONS
During Muscle-Shortening Phase	
In Movement	
▪ Rotating the trunk (or even the hips) to the right or left.	▪ Maintaining a strict side-to-side movement.
▪ Minimally raising the trunk.	▪ Raising the trunk as high as possible (30°–45° past the neutral position).
▪ Immediately lowering the trunk after reaching the midpoint.	▪ Briefly holding the squeezed side (incorporating an isometric contraction) at the midpoint to work the quadratus lumborum, a deep side muscle.
In Stillness	
▪ Bending the lower knee, which engages the hip muscles by shifting the pelvis.	▪ Keeping the knees straight to ensure that the hip joint muscles stabilize the pelvic girdle and that the trunk and spinal muscles do the work.
During Muscle-Lengthening Phase	
In Movement	
▪ Minimally lowering the trunk.	▪ Lowering the trunk almost as far as it can go (thereby placing the targeted muscles on maximum stretch).

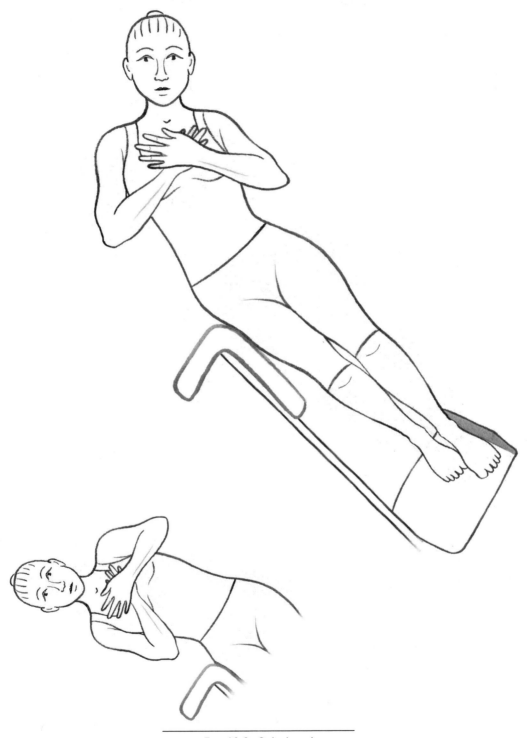

Fig. 10.3. Side bend

Ab Curl

Decline Abdominal Bench

Joint movements: lumbar flexion
Lumbar flexion is forward movement of the thorax toward the pelvis.

Muscles most involved in joint movements: rectus abdominis, external oblique (on both sides), and internal oblique (on both sides)

POSITIONING

1. Bend your knees to hook your feet under the foot brace as you lie on your back on the decline bench.
2. Lightly clasp your hands behind your neck with your arms perpendicular to your head.
3. Arch your lower back (pre-stretching the abdominals increases the amount of force generated).
   Note: To increase the difficulty, increase the angle of decline, hold a plate at your chest, or hold a plate behind your neck.

MOVEMENT

1. Curl your trunk up so your sternum (breastbone) moves closer to your pubis (pubic bone). As your trunk rises, contract your stomach, flatten your lumbar spine, and tilt your pelvis backward.
2. Briefly hold the position.
3. Return to the starting position.

COMMON ERRORS	CORRECTIONS
During Muscle-Shortening Phase	
In Movement	
■ Breathing in (which distends the stomach).	■ Breathing out (which flattens the stomach).
■ Lifting up with a jerky movement (which puts undue pressure on the lower spine).	■ Curling up gradually.
■ Immediately beginning to lower the back after reaching the midpoint.	Incorporating an isometric contraction at the midpoint to work the transversus abdominis, the deep abdominal muscle.
In Stillness	
■ Pulling on the head.	■ Keeping the head aligned with the torso.
■ Raising the torso more than 30°–45° off the bench.	■ Limiting the raising of the torso to 30°–45° off the bench (a higher raise recruits the psoas muscle, a hip joint flexor).
During Muscle-Lengthening Phase	
In Movement	
■ Flopping back down.	■ Curling down slowly and with control.

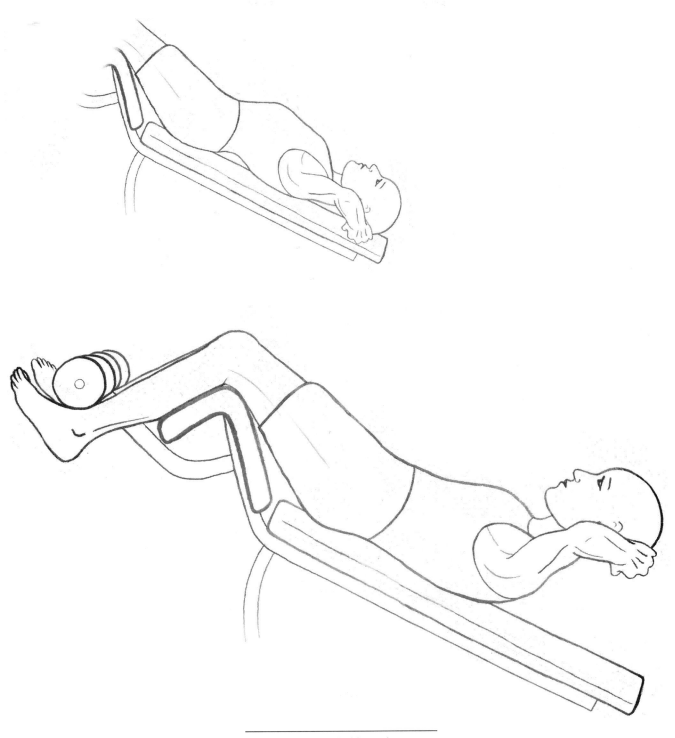

Fig. 10.4. Ab curl

Seated Twist

Cam Lumbar Rotation Machine

Joint movements: lumbar rotation
Lumbar rotation is the twisting movement of the thorax to one side.

Muscles most involved in joint movements: external oblique (on one side) and internal oblique (on the opposite side)

POSITIONING

1. Adjust the range-of-motion setting of the upper pads to one side.
2. Grasp the handgrips.
3. Sit with your chest against the upper pads. Squeeze your knees against the lower pads.
4. Slightly rotate your trunk.

MOVEMENT

1. Twist your trunk to the opposite side.
2. Return to the starting position.
3. After completing the set, repeat the action with the other side.

COMMON ERRORS	CORRECTIONS
During Muscle-Shortening Phase	
In Movement	
■ Twisting quickly. (When seated, the lumbar discs are already compressed 40% more than while standing; moving quickly creates a shearing force, risking injury.)	■ Twisting slowly and with control.
In Stillness	
■ Initiating the movement with external rotation of the upper arm (posterior deltoids, infraspinatus, and teres minor), retraction of the shoulder blade (rhomboids), abduction of the hip (hip abductors), and external rotation of the leg (deep lateral hip rotators).	■ Keeping the chest, shoulders, and upper back aligned with the spine and keeping the hips and legs facing forward.
During Muscle-Lengthening Phase	
In Movement	
■ Untwisting too quickly.	■ Returning to the starting position slowly and with control.

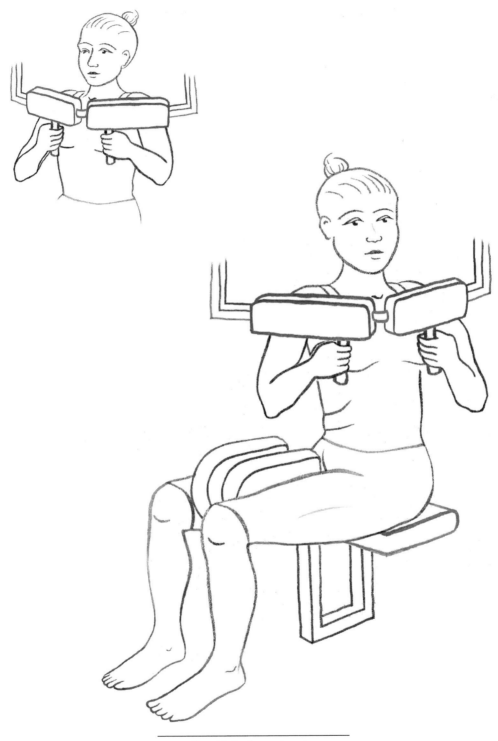

Fig. 10.5. Seated twist

Neck Bends

Plate-Loaded Neck Machine

Joint movements: cervical extension, flexion, and lateral flexion
Cervical extension is backward movement of the head away from the chest. Cervical flexion is forward movement of the head toward the chest. Cervical lateral flexion is sideways movement of the head toward the shoulder.

Muscles most involved in joint movements: extension—splenius cervicis, splenius capitis, erector spinae, and upper trapezius (on both sides); flexion—sternocleidomastoid (on both sides); lateral flexion—sternocleidomastoid, splenius cervicis, splenius capitis, and erector spinae (on one side)

POSITIONING

1. To work the neck all the way around—in all four directions—use a four-way neck machine, adjusting the head pad, the seat, and/or your position. Sit down, and grip the handles. For extension, place the back of your head on the pad. For flexion, place the front of your head on the pad. For lateral flexion, place the side of your head on the pad.
2. For each exercise, slightly press your head against the pad, using only your neck.

MOVEMENT

1. For extension, press your head backward against the pad as far as possible, using only your neck. For flexion, press your head forward against the pad as far as possible, using only your neck. For lateral flexion, press your head sideways against the pad as far as possible, using only your neck.
2. After each movement, return to the starting position.

COMMON ERRORS	CORRECTIONS
During Muscle-Shortening Phase	
In Movement	
■ Limiting the range of motion of the neck movements.	■ Moving the head as far as possible in each direction.
In Stillness	
■ Allowing secondary muscles of the trunk to initiate the movement.	■ Isolating the neck muscles by keeping the trunk immobile (chest up, back erect, and sides straight).
■ Lifting off the seat.	■ Remaining secure on the seat.
During Muscle-Lengthening Phase	
In Movement	
■ Letting the neck snap back.	■ Returning to the original position using a slow and controlled movement.

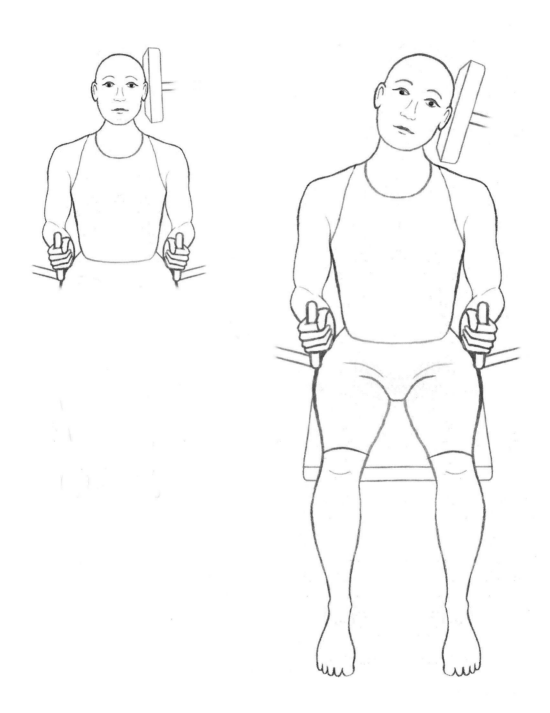

Fig. 10.6. Left lateral neck bend

11

EXERCISES FOR THE HIP JOINT AND PELVIC GIRDLE

The hip joint is formed by the smooth, spherical surface of the head of the thighbone (femur), the longest bone in the body, snugly fitting into the deep cavity of the pelvis. (The hip joint is more stable, and therefore less mobile, than the shoulder joint.)

The muscles that originate on the pelvis and spinal column and cross the hip joint are the iliopsoas and other muscles that insert on the front of the thighbone; the gluteus maximus, hamstrings, and other muscles that insert on the back of the thighbone; and the hip abductors and hip adductors that insert on the sides of the thighbone.

The hip joint is a ball-and-socket joint, which permits these muscles to produce horizontal, side-to-side, and front-to-back movements of the upper leg:

- turning the leg toward the midline (45° of internal rotation) and turning the leg away from the midline (50° of external rotation);
- from the raised side position, sweeping the leg across the midline (65° to 80° of adduction), and raising the leg from the side of the body out to the side (45° to 50° degrees of abduction);
- and, with the knee bent, raising the leg forward and up (130° of flexion) and, from the bent-knee-raised position, moving the leg down and back behind the body (150° to 170° degrees of extension).

At the back of the pelvic girdle, the sacrum fits between the two pelvic bones to form the sacroiliac joints. Because the sacroiliac joints are immobile in most adults, muscles of other parts of the body as well as those of the pelvis produce front-to-back movement of the pelvis:

- rotating the pelvis backward to flatten the curvature of the lower back (posterior pelvic tilt), and rotating the pelvis forward to accentuate the curvature of the lower back (anterior pelvic tilt).

Hip movements performed against resistance strengthen the thick hip joint muscles to provide stability and to promote mobility (such as walking with a spring in the step).

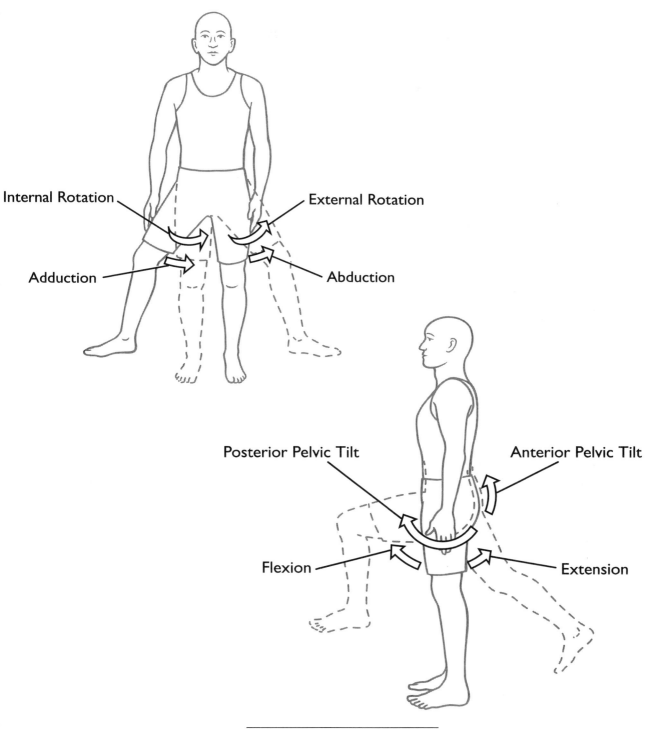

Internal Rotation

External Rotation

Adduction

Abduction

Posterior Pelvic Tilt

Anterior Pelvic Tilt

Flexion

Extension

Fig. 11.1. Hip joint movements: internal rotation and external rotation, adduction
and abduction, and flexion and extension
Pelvic girdle movements: posterior pelvic tilt and anterior pelvic tilt

Bent-Leg Hip Extension

Cable Crossover Machine

Joint movements: hip joint extension and external rotation

Hip joint extension is movement of the upper leg straight backward and upward. Hip joint external rotation is the rotary movement of the upper leg around its longitudinal axis away from the midline.

Muscles most involved in joint movements: gluteus maximus

POSITIONING

1. Place one of the pulleys in the lowest position. Attach an ankle strap to the pulley, and wrap the strap's cuff around the ankle of your moving leg. Grasp the bar with both hands.
2. As you step back with your supporting leg, tilt forward (with your back straight).
3. Fully bend your moving knee (you should be positioned far enough back so that your bent knee doesn't hit the machine).

MOVEMENT

1. Keeping your upper body and supporting leg motionless, bring your moving leg back while simultaneously outwardly rotating it at the thigh.
2. Return to the starting position.
3. After the completing the set, repeat the action with your other leg.
   Note: To decrease the difficulty, extend your hip with the aid of your hamstrings by straightening your leg as you move it back.

COMMON ERRORS	CORRECTIONS
During Muscle-Shortening Phase	
In Movement	
■ Pulling the leg back as far as possible by arching the lower back (which strains the lumbar spine by creating excessive extension).	■ Bringing the leg back only slightly behind the trunk (to prevent the pelvis from tilting forward and the lower back from arching).
In Stillness	
■ Bending the trunk (to use momentum to kick the leg back).	■ Maintaining a straight back (while the body itself is tilted).
■ Twisting the trunk to the outside (to cheat on the leg rotation).	■ Keeping the trunk facing forward (while outwardly rotating the leg).
■ Straightening the moving leg.	■ Keeping the moving leg bent.
During Muscle-Lengthening Phase	
In Movement	
■ Swinging the leg forward without fully bending the knee.	■ Bending the knee fully (to maximally stretch the hip extensors).

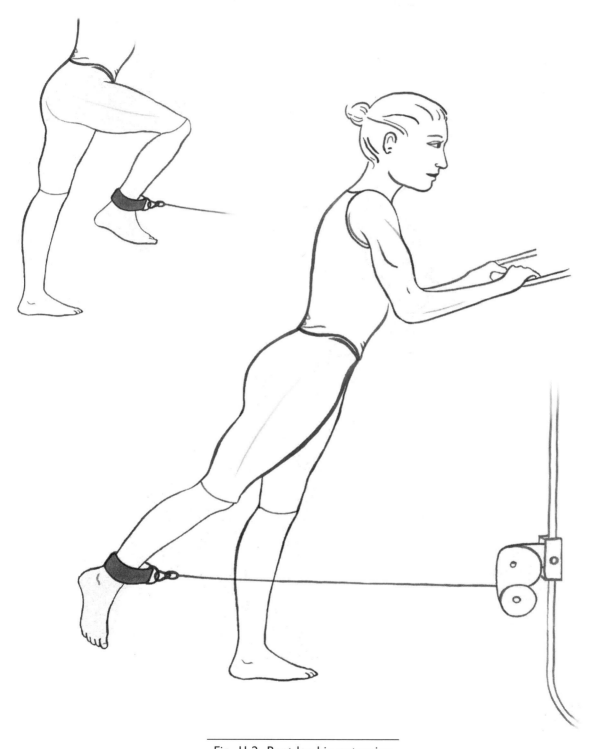

Fig. 11.2. Bent-leg hip extension

Hanging Knee Raise
Captain's Chair

Joint movements: hip joint flexion and external rotation

Hip joint flexion is movement of the upper leg straight forward and upward. Hip joint external rotation is the rotary movement of the upper leg around its longitudinal axis away from the midline.

Muscles most involved in joint movements: iliopsoas, rectus femoris, and pectineus

POSITIONING

1. Facing outward, step up into the frame. Grab the upright handles, rest your forearms on the chair arms, and dangle your legs close together with your feet pointed slightly inward.
2. To prevent stress on the lumbar spine (where the psoas originates), tilt your pelvis posteriorly (flatten your lower back), and brace your abdominal muscles.
3. Slightly lift your legs (where the iliopsoas inserts at their top).

MOVEMENT

1. Slowly lift your legs as high as you can with your knees bent. Simultaneously, powerfully contract your abdominals to prevent lower back strain (they pull on the front of the pelvis, thus aiding the flattening of the back), and rotate your legs slightly outward.

   Note: To increase the difficulty, lift with your legs straight. The long resistance arm of straightened legs requires greater muscular force to move than bent legs.
2. Return to the starting position.

COMMON ERRORS	CORRECTIONS
During Muscle-Shortening Phase	
In Movement	
■ Thrusting the knees up by tilting the pelvis anteriorly and arching the back, causing lower back strain.	■ Pressing the lower back to the back of the machine by mightily tightening the abdomen to prevent the pelvis from tilting anteriorly and prevent the lower back from extending.
In Stillness	
■ Rocking the head.	■ Keeping the head steady.
During Muscle-Lengthening Phase	
In Movement	
■ Lowering the legs too quickly.	■ Lowering the legs moderately slowly.
■ Bending the knees.	■ Keeping the legs straight.

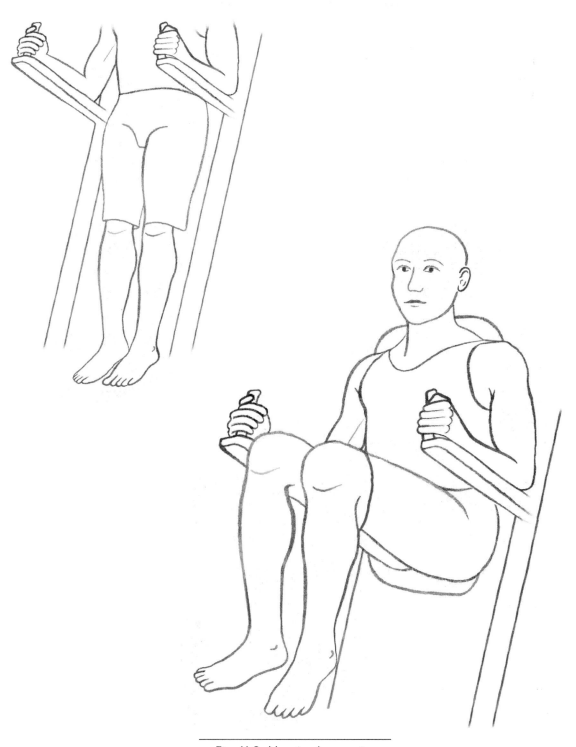

Fig. 11.3. Hanging knee raise

Hip Abduction

Cable Crossover Machine

Joint movements: hip joint abduction
Hip joint abduction is movement of the upper leg away from the midline toward the side.

Muscles most involved in joint movements: gluteus medius, gluteus minimus, and tensor fasciae latae

POSITIONING

1. Place one of the pulleys about 6 inches from the lowest position. Attach an ankle strap to the pulley, and wrap the strap's cuff around the ankle of your moving leg. Grasp the bar with the hand that's on the side of your supporting leg.
2. Stand sideways to the machine with your supporting leg (on a plate to keep the moving leg from hitting the floor) near the pulley and slightly behind your moving leg.
3. Slightly lift your moving leg. Don't lean to the side any more than you need to for standing on one leg.

MOVEMENT

1. Keeping the upper body motionless and erect and the supporting leg fixed, lift the moving leg straight out to the side (away from the body) as high as possible.
2. Return to the starting position.
3. After completing the set, repeat the action with the other leg.
   Note: To develop the internal and external rotation actions of the targeted muscles, slightly turn the toes inward or outward during the movement.

COMMON ERRORS	CORRECTIONS
During Muscle-Shortening Phase	
In Movement	
■ Insufficiently lifting the leg up.	■ Bringing the leg up to the full range of motion (about 35°).
In Stillness	
■ Leaning the trunk to the opposite of the leg movement (to gain more leverage and possibly use momentum to increase the leg's range of motion).	■ Keeping the trunk erect and motionless (to isolate the targeted muscles).
■ Rotating the pelvis anteriorly.	■ Preventing the forward and downward tilting of the pelvis by tightening the abdomen (thereby pulling the pelvis up in front).
During Muscle-Lengthening Phase	
In Movement	
■ Lowering the leg too quickly.	■ Lowering the leg moderately slowly.

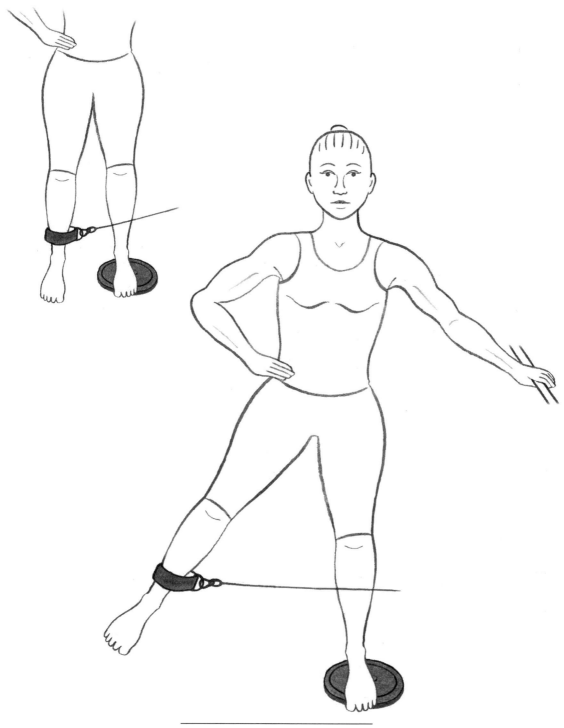

Fig. 11.4. Hip abduction

Hip Adduction

Hip Adductor Cam Machine

Joint movements: hip joint adduction

Hip joint adduction is movement of the upper leg toward the midline from the side.

Muscles most involved in joint movements: adductor magnus, adductor longus, adductor brevis, pectineus, and gracilis

POSITIONING

1. Pull the release handle to open the leg units to a challenging width
2. Straddle the seat by standing on the foot pegs. With your buttocks against the backrest, place your knees to the kneepads. Slide down onto the seat while pushing the kneepads with your knees and hands.
3. Adjust your feet on the foot pegs to create a 90° angle between your lower and upper legs. Grasp the handgrips. Sit tall with your back pressed against the backrest. **Note:** To avoid an overstretching injury, start with your legs comfortably apart and gradually widen them over time.

MOVEMENT

1. Use your inner thighs to initiate bringing your legs together.
2. Return to the starting position.
3. To exit the machine, press your hands to the front of your legs and scooch straight up until you're straddling the seat by standing on the foot pegs. Step off to one side. **Note:** To mildly develop the internal rotation actions of the pectineus and gracilis muscles, turn the legs slightly inward (with the feet somewhat pigeon-toed). To mildly develop the external rotation actions of adductor brevis and adductor magnus, turn the legs slightly outward (with the feet somewhat splayed).

COMMON ERRORS	CORRECTIONS
During Muscle-Shortening Phase	
In Movement	
▪ Stopping the leg movement before the kneepads touch.	▪ Moving the legs until the kneepads touch.
In Stillness	
▪ Arching the back.	▪ Keeping the back against the seat.
▪ Rotating the pelvis anteriorly.	▪ Preventing the forward tilting of the pelvis by contracting the abdomen.
During Muscle-Lengthening Phase	
In Movement	
▪ Letting the legs snap back.	▪ Controlling the outward leg movement.
▪ Failing to return the legs all the way to the starting position.	▪ Moving the legs out enough so that the lifted weights nearly return to the weight stack.

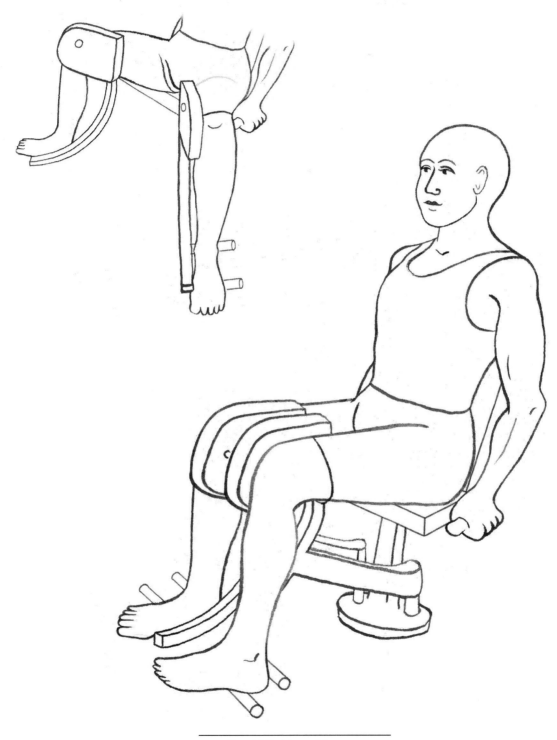

Fig. 11.5. Hip adduction

12

EXERCISES
FOR THE KNEE JOINT

The knee joint, the largest joint in the body, is complex: not only does the thighbone (femur) connect to the shinbone (tibia) but also to the kneecap (patella). The quadriceps muscles, which originate at the front of the pelvis and thighbone, attach to the kneecap tendon, which, in turn, crosses the knee joint to the front of the shinbone; the hamstring muscles, which originate at the back of the pelvis, cross the knee joint to insert on the back of the shinbone.

Although the knee undergoes some rotation, the knee joint is primarily a hinge joint, which permits its muscles to produce only front-to-back movements of the lower leg:

■ from the 90° bent-knee position, straightening the knee (90° of extension), an action of the quadriceps (the kneecap, a floating bone, serves as a pulley for the quadriceps in knee extension), and, from the resting position, bending the knee back toward the buttocks (120° to 130° of flexion), an action of the hamstrings.

In conjunction with the hip and ankle joints, the knee joint holds up the body and moves the body; these combined functions place considerable stress on the knee joint. Knee joint movements performed against resistance strengthen the powerful knee joint muscles to prevent knee injuries and to make everyday weight-bearing activities (such as standing while waiting in line) and locomotion (such as climbing stairs) easier.

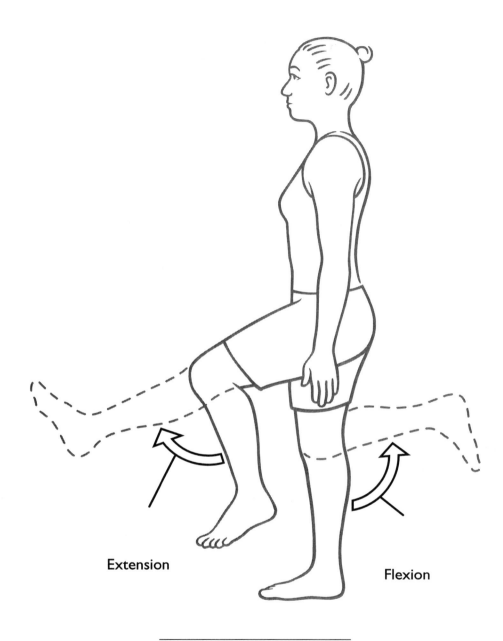

Extension

Flexion

Fig. 12.1. Knee joint movements: extension and flexion

Prone Knee Curl

Cam Prone Knee Curl Machine

Joint movements: knee joint flexion

Knee joint flexion is movement of the lower leg from a straightened to a bent position, thereby decreasing the angle between the back of the thigh and the lower leg.

Muscles most involved in joint movements: hamstrings, biceps femoris, semimembranosus, and semitendinosus

POSITIONING

1. Adjust the roller so it will be at the back of your ankles.
2. Lie face down on the angled bench. (The angle flexes your hip joints, allowing your upper hamstrings to stretch and thus freeing your lower hamstrings at the knee joints to initiate the action on their own.) Place your knees over the edge (unsupported) and the back of your ankles against the underside of the roller.
3. Hold the handgrips.
4. Slightly lift your lower legs.

MOVEMENT

1. Bend your knees to bring your lower legs toward the back of your thighs (between 90° and 130°).
2. Return to the starting position.

   Note: To increase the difficulty, point your feet away from your shins, reducing the involvement of the gastrocnemius, a calf muscle that crosses the knee. To decrease the difficulty, point your feet toward your shins, engaging the gastrocnemius.

COMMON ERRORS	CORRECTIONS
During Muscle-Shortening Phase	
In Movement	
▪ Flinging the lower legs up by kicking the heels back.	▪ Raising the lower legs moderately slowly and with control.
▪ Bringing the lower legs up to less than a vertical position.	▪ Bending the knees until the calves are at least slightly past the vertical position.
In Stillness	
▪ Hyperextending the lower back and raising the hips and thighs (thereby initiating a thrusting movement of the legs).	▪ Keeping the lower back in a neutral position by co-contracting the abdominal and lower back muscles.
	▪ Keeping the hips and thighs in contact with the bench.
During Muscle-Lengthening Phase	
In Movement	
▪ Letting the lower legs flop down.	▪ Lowering the lower legs with control.

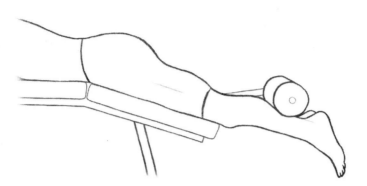

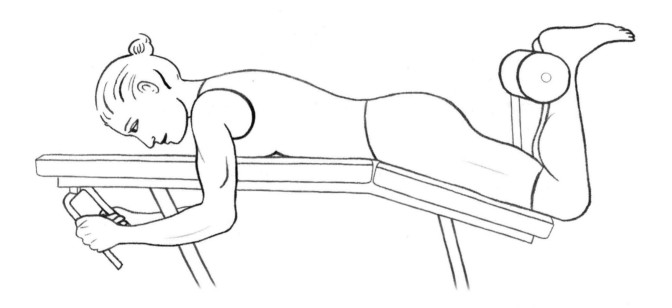

Fig. 12.2. Prone knee curl

Knee Extension

Cam Knee Extension Machine

Joint movements: knee joint extension

Knee joint extension is movement of the lower leg from a bent to a straightened position, thereby increasing the angle between the back of the thigh and the lower leg.

Muscles most involved in joint movements: quadriceps: rectus femoris, vastus medialis, vastus intermedius, and vastus lateralis

POSITIONING

1. Adjust the back, seat, and resistance pad so that when you sit down, you can lean back and place your knees just over the edge of the seat and the front of your ankles against the pad. Square your legs (your knee joint is at a 90° angle).
2. Hold the handgrips, and slightly lift your legs, placing your shins in front of your thighs.
   Note: Over time, gradually increase the range of motion until you're starting with your shins slightly under your thighs.

MOVEMENT

1. Lift your lower legs to full or nearly full extension.
   Note: Fully extending your legs (to 180° of extension) is critical for helping to maintain a proper line of pull for the kneecap and aiding in knee stability, because the group of muscle fibers of the vastus medialis that counterbalances the stronger vastus lateralis primarily contracts during the last 10°–20° of knee extension.
2. Return to the starting position.

COMMON ERRORS	CORRECTIONS
During Muscle-Shortening Phase	
In Movement	
▪ Flinging the legs up.	▪ Raising the legs moderately slowly.
▪ Limiting the range of motion to less than optimal extension.	▪ Bringing the knees up to a locked or nearly locked position.
In Stillness	
▪ Lunging.	▪ Keeping the back against the seat. (Bending forward reduces the effectiveness of the rectus femoris as a knee extensor, shifting the work primarily to the other three muscles.)
▪ Thrusting the legs up with the hips and lower back	
During Muscle-Lengthening Phase	
In Movement	
▪ Letting the legs flop down.	▪ Lowering the legs slowly and with control.

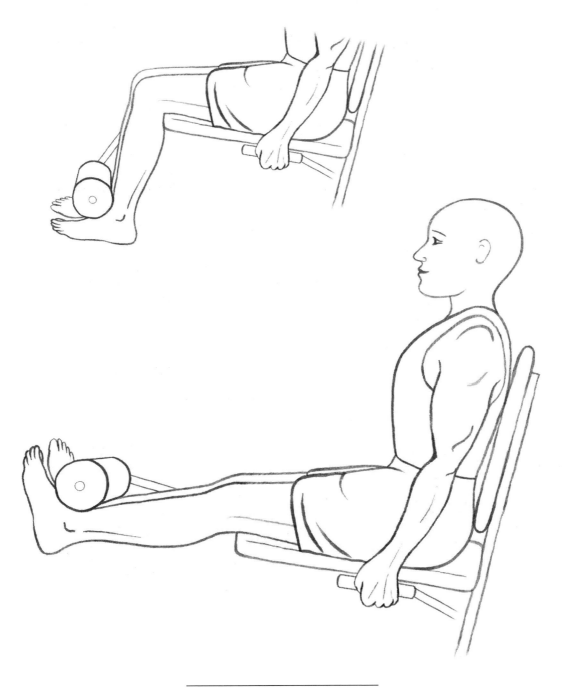

Fig. 12.3. Knee extension

13

EXERCISES
FOR THE ANKLE JOINT

The ankle joint tightly connects the two bones of the lower leg (tibia and fibula) to the small bone (talus) that sits above the heel bone of the foot.

The gastrocnemius, which originates on the back of the upper and lower legs, and the soleus, which originates on the back of the lower leg, insert on the Achilles tendon, which crosses the ankle joint to connect the two calf muscles to the heel; and tibialis anterior, extensor digitorum longus, and extensor hallucis longus, which originate on the front of the lower leg, cross the ankle joint to insert on the foot.

The ankle joint is a hinge joint, which permits these muscles to produce only front-to-back movement of the foot:

- raising the ankle and foot upward toward the shin (15° to 20° of flexion, or dorsiflexion), an action primarily of tibialis anterior, and pointing the ankle and foot downward or raising the heel upward (45° to 50° degrees of extension, or plantar flexion), an action of the gastrocnemius and soleus.

Unlike most mammals, whose weight is distributed among four feet, humans stand and move on two feet. The ankle joint, in conjunction with the knee and hip joints, has a double function: bearing the weight of the body (support) and moving the body (propulsion). The ankle joint movements performed against resistance strengthen the lower legs to prevent shin splints, cramps, and other painful calf conditions; to make everyday activities that require support and movement easier; and to propel the body upward and forward in sports activities (such as jumping and running in basketball).

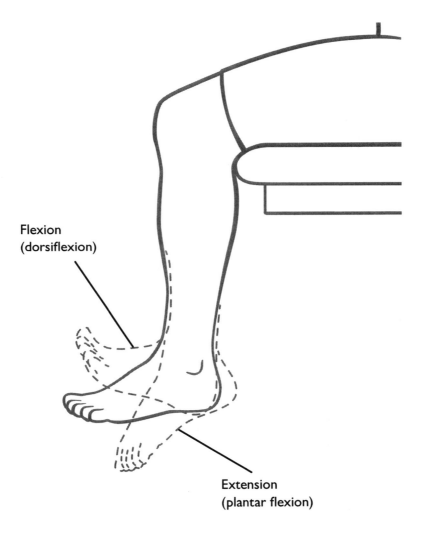

Flexion (dorsiflexion)

Extension (plantar flexion)

Fig. 13.1. Ankle joint movements: flexion and extension

Standing Heel Raise

Plate-Loaded Standing Calf Machine

Joint movements: ankle joint extension (plantar flexion)

Ankle joint extension (paradoxically called plantar flexion) is movement of the foot by raising the heel or pointing the toes downward, thereby increasing the angle between the bottom of the foot (the plantar surface) and the shin.

Muscles most involved in joint movements: gastrocnemius and soleus

POSITIONING

1. As you step onto the platform with your feet shoulder-width apart, bend your knees, and place your shoulders under the lever pads (in a squatting position). Place the balls of your feet squarely on the platform (with your feet facing straight ahead).
2. Pressing up on the lever pads, straighten your legs to assume an erect (not hunched over) standing position.
3. Lower your heels.

MOVEMENT

1. Press off the inside balls of your feet to lift your heels.
2. Return to the starting position.

COMMON ERRORS	CORRECTIONS
During Muscle-Shortening Phase	
In Movement	
▪ Bouncing up.	▪ Raising the heels moderately slowly and with control to avoid bouncing.
▪ Pressing off the outside balls of the feet and the last three toes.	▪ Pressing off the inside balls of the feet.
▪ Raising the heels to less than the maximum range of motion.	▪ Raising the heels as high as possible.
In Stillness	
▪ Bending the knees (thereby involving the gastrocnemius less and the soleus more).	▪ Keeping the knees straight (maintaining the full involvement of the gastrocnemius).
▪ Pushing the hips forward.	▪ Holding the back in a neutral position with the head erect.
During Muscle-Lengthening Phase	
In Movement	
▪ Lowering the heels quickly (thus letting gravity overpower the movement).	▪ Lowering the heels moderately slowly and with control (to resist the pull of gravity).

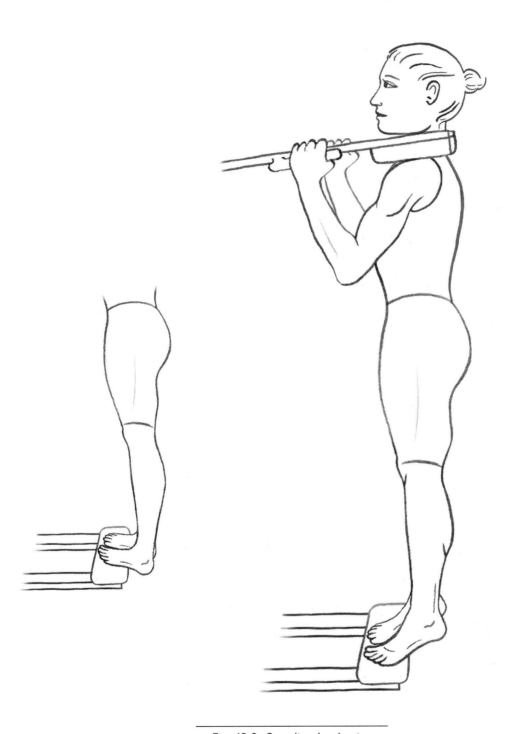

Fig. I3.2. Standing heel raise

Seated Heel Raise

Plate-Loaded Seated Calf Machine

Joint movements: ankle joint extension (plantar flexion)
Ankle joint extension (paradoxically called plantar flexion) is movement of the foot by raising the heel or pointing the toes downward, thereby increasing the angle between the bottom of the foot (the plantar surface) and the shin.

Muscles most involved in joint movements: soleus

POSITIONING

1. Sit on the seat with your legs bent at a 90° angle and the resistance pad nearly resting on the top of your front thighs. Place the balls of your feet on the block, with your heels free to move.
2. Pull the release handle to lower the weights. The resistance pad should now be firmly resting on your front thighs.
3. Lower your heels.

MOVEMENT

1. Press off the inside balls of your feet to lift your heels.
2. Return to the starting position.

COMMON ERRORS	CORRECTIONS
During Muscle-Shortening Phase	
In Movement	
■ Bouncing the resistance by quickly raising the heels.	■ Raising the heels moderately slowly and with control to avoid bouncing.
■ Pressing off the outside balls of the feet and the last three toes.	■ Pressing off the inside balls of the feet.
■ Raising the heels to less than the maximum range of motion.	■ Raising the heels as high as possible.
In Stillness	
■ Arching the back.	■ Holding the back taut (with its natural curves) by co-tightening the abdomen and lower back.
■ Leaning forward.	■ Keeping the trunk erect.
During Muscle-Lengthening Phase	
In Movement	
■ Lowering the heels to less than the maximum range of motion.	■ Lowering the heels nearly as low as possible.
■ Lowering the heels quickly (thus letting gravity overpower the movement).	■ Lowering the heels moderately slowly and with control (to resist the pull of gravity).

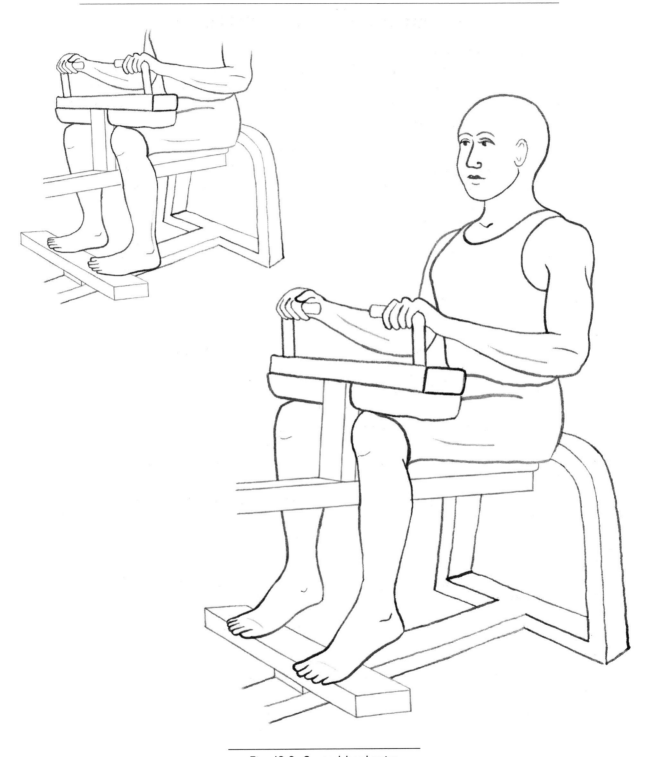

Fig. 13.3. Seated heel raise

Weighted Toe Raise

Ankle Strap and Dumbbell

Joint movements: ankle joint flexion (dorsiflexion)
Ankle joint flexion (called dorsiflexion) is movement of the foot by pointing the toes upward, thereby decreasing the angle between the top of the foot (the dorsal surface) and the shin.

Muscles most involved in joint movements: tibialis anterior, extensor digitorum longus, and peroneus tertius

POSITIONING

1. Wrap an ankle strap around a dumbbell handle. Tie one end of a cord to the D-ring attachment of the ankle strap. Tie the other end of the cord around your foot.
2. Prop yourself up on a high seat with your leg bent at a 90° angle.
3. Point your foot downward.

MOVEMENT

1. Raise the top of your foot toward your shin.
2. Return to the starting position.

COMMON ERRORS	CORRECTIONS
During Muscle-Shortening Phase	
In Movement	
▪ Quickly raising the top of the foot.	▪ Raising the top of the foot moderately slowly and with control.
▪ Raising the top of the foot to less than the maximum range of motion.	▪ Raising the top of the foot as high as possible.
In Stillness	
▪ Swinging the lower leg up.	▪ Keeping the lower leg vertical.
During Muscle-Lengthening Phase	
In Movement	
▪ Lowering the top of the foot to less than the maximum range of motion.	▪ Lowering the top of the foot nearly as low as possible.
▪ Lowering the top of the foot too quickly.	▪ Lowering the top of the foot moderately slowly and with control.
In Stillness	
▪ Swinging the lower leg back.	▪ Keeping the knee at a right angle.

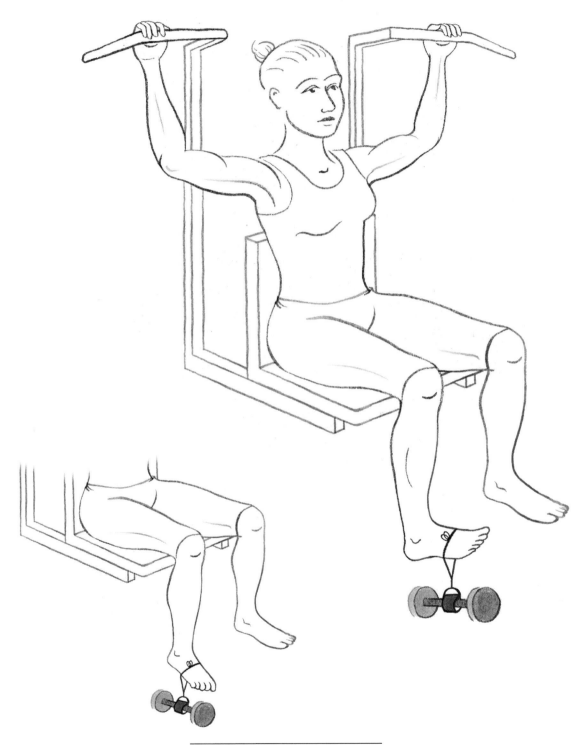

Fig. 13.4. Weighted toe raise

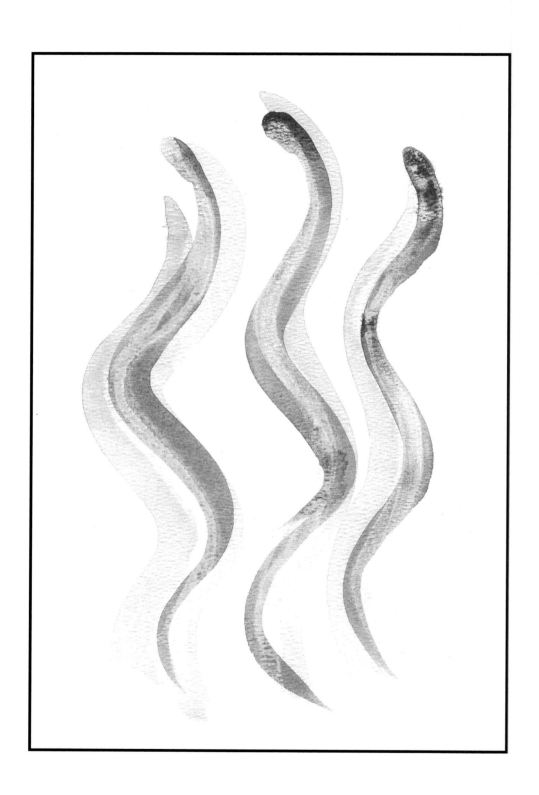

PART THREE

. . . .

Meditations

We're rarely in touch with the true nature of our existence. How could it be otherwise? Most of the time we're too busy just getting through the day. It may take some occurrence out of the ordinary or an ordinary but striking occurrence to interrupt our preoccupation with the necessities of daily life, compelling us to reflect on our existence. We've all had experiences of this sort. Some of my own that come to mind are, after a prolonged, bitter argument with my wife, a reconciliation brought about by mutual apology and forgiveness; being suddenly overwhelmed by the beauty of drifting clouds seen when stepping out of the house; the loss of my best friend in an automobile accident while he was vacationing in Ireland, leaving me with an unending sense of the fleetingness of life.

The apprehension of our existence can also be systematically cultivated: it may be manifested as an insight during a religious rite that's part of a long-established pattern of observance or a hard-won realization in a psychotherapy session after a lengthy period of treatment or an opening up during a sustained, disciplined meditative practice.

Like these examples, the comprehensions that take place during a weight-resistance yoga session happen over time during a designated period of time set aside to cultivate them. They occur not through talk or prayer or concentration on the lotus of the heart, however, but through the experience of the body during motions against resistance.

In the *Yoga Sutras,* Patanjali explains that access to a deepened sense of existence—what he calls liberation of self—can be achieved by a series of eight steps. These steps are *yama* (observing certain restraints), *niyama* (observing certain disciplines), *asana* (performing exercises), *pranayama* (breathing rhythmically), *pratyahara* (calming the senses), *dharana* (concentrating on aspects of bodily movement), *dhyana* (grasping the body—in its stillness, stability, and movement—as a whole), and *samadhi* (all concern with the self disregarded, comprehending reality that's hidden beneath everyday life. In weight-resistance yoga (as in some recent expressions of weight-surrender yoga), all the steps are incorporated into the embodied experience of the exercise practice.

By following this eight-step path, we transmute common strengthening exercises (usually performed with dumbbells and barbells and machines) into an ascetic discipline by which Being—the fullness of the permanent—is disclosed to us, as it opens up around us.

MEDITATIONS ON THE SHOULDER JOINT

■ **On Expressiveness—Introduction to the Shoulder Joint**

The shoulder joint is a very weak bony arrangement. But it's exactly the fragileness of this joint that allows it to move so freely—and allows the arms to be so expressive.

■ **On Wholeness—Lat Pulldown**

Their great length and breadth are what give the lats their powerful pulling action on the arms. Which is why having strong lats appeals to our fantasies of adventure: dangling from a ledge, we would use these mighty muscles to hoist ourselves up to safety.

■ **On Gravity—Shoulder Press**

When Zeus defeated Atlas in battle he forced Atlas to support the heavens on his shoulders forever. Curiously, many works of art show Atlas bearing the weight of Earth instead. Perhaps this is because we mortals so often feel the burden of "carrying the world on our shoulders."

■ **On Right Tension—Seated Low Row**

The seated low row is one of the most inviting exercises in the gym, because it mirrors rowing a boat—for most of us, a seemingly pleasurable long-ago pastime. By turns, we pull back on the oars and let ourselves be pulled forward—rhythmic motions against and with the water.

■ **On Harmony—Standing High Row**

Around 1490 Leonardo da Vinci completed his famous pen-and-ink drawing of the naked figure with perfect proportions—*Vitruvian Man*. In practicing weight-resistance yoga, we don't achieve perfect bodily proportions, but we do forge a body that's configured to the harmony of its own unique skeletal structure.

On Expressiveness
Introduction to the Shoulder Joint

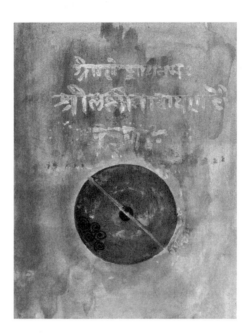

*With steady calm and half-closed eyes fixed on the tip of the nose,
the yogi attains the state wherein he can see the light which is all.
What is the use of more talk?*

—Svatmarama, *The Hatha Yoga Pradipika*

The shoulder joint is formed by the articulation of the oval head of the upper arm bone (humerus) and the socket (glenoid fossa) of the shoulder blade (scapula). It's a very weak bony arrangement: the shoulder blade cavity is so shallow it can only receive a small area of the head of the arm bone. Which is why it's easy as pie to yank an arm out of its socket. But it's exactly this fragileness that makes the shoulder joint so freely movable. And it's this great range and variety of movement that makes possible the expressiveness of the arms. To a great extent, the arms move as we please—and, sometimes, as we don't please.

There's no denying the incomparable expressiveness of the face. But, as Mabel E. Todd, a pioneer of understanding body alignment as a function of mechanical principles, noted, "A casual world over-emphasizes the face.

Memory likes to recall the whole body"—of which the arms are an integral part.[1] I remember three generations of women: at our first meeting, my mother-in-law, in her sixties, turning sideways and placing her arms akimbo to show off her shapely figure; my wife squatting down and extending her arms to our old arthritic dog, who pokily slips and slides toward her; my daughter, as a teenager, crossing her arms to indicate disengagement. You, I'm sure, have your own album of such recollections.

Although we're generally free to express our emotions with our arms (how free may depend on our temperament, ethnicity, sex, or other determinants), we're also asked to restrain our arms, and we comply. It's part of being grown up. We no longer flop them in frustration, or make windmill circles as we walk down the street, or place them between our legs and press them together with our thighs (at least, not in public). In some ways, our humeral vocabulary, it might be said, becomes more somber. And it's equally true that sometimes our arms, like unruly children, get away from us and misbehave, as any of us know who have intemperately embraced someone or shaken our arms in anger.

When carrying out weightlifting exercises, our arms don't express emotions or ideas. (Sometimes it's hard to separate the articulateness of the arms from their loquacious extensions, the hands. But because our hands are muted by their grip on a handle or bar during shoulder joint exercises, the expressiveness of our arms is further inhibited.) They merely have a prosaic function providing strength.

But not in the way many people think. What appears to be an exercise for arm muscles is often an exercise for back, shoulder, or chest muscles. Muscles originating on the torso—the deltoids, pectoralis, and latissimus dorsi (or "delts," "pecs," and "lats," as they're called in the gym), as well as other muscles—cross over the shoulder joints to insert on the arms. The muscles of the arms, assisted by the hands, act as servants to these mostly bigger muscles by moving the weights. But it's the torso muscles that apply most of the force and receive most of the strength gain in shoulder joint exercises.

The success of shoulder joint exercises depends, in part, on the exactness of the trajectory of our arms. Commonly, weightlifting movements are performed carelessly: either hurriedly by thrusting and yanking or in a wobbly and desultory manner. They express impatience and boredom. What distinguishes weight-resistance yoga arm movement during shoulder joint exercises is that the trajectory of the arms is controlled, carefully prescribed, and realized with an economy of motion—thereby removing all emotion.

That's why weight-resistance yoga shoulder joint movements closely resemble the semaphore system of signaling, in which the movements of the arms are geometric and abstract. All weight-resistance yoga movements partake of this formality; but it's most apparent in shoulder joint exercises exactly because the arms are so expressive under ordinary circumstances.

Weight-resistance yoga practice is a form of tapas, or austerity. (The root of the word *tapas* means "heat" or "to make hot." Sometimes meaning "being ardent," "having burning desire," or simply "burning desire," *tapas* may also mean "austerity"—an action that purifies the body by "burning up impurities.") It's a vow of silence applied to the *body*. The body is not only struck speechless, though; it's also stripped of its individuality, of its personality. Every body that perfectly performs a weightlifting exercise utters the same language, or rather, is reduced to the same muteness. No wonder the impassive movements of weight-resistance yoga make us anxious at first!

But if we can bear this almost death-like absence of gestures (and of the other corporeal manifestations of our mind stuff: facial expressions and idiosyncratic posture and gait)—if we can bear this elimination, you might say, of our humanity—what happens, strangely enough, is that in the very precision and economy of movement that results from suppressing the body's everyday expression of emotions, the body—perhaps especially the arms—finds expression after all: a kind of calm and quiet.

This transformation helps make it possible for us to breathe evenly and rhythmically, and then to observe and control the feelings and thoughts that drift along in our mind like the debris of a house swept up in a flood. And on those days when we're blessed, these pared down and controlled movements become a prelude to the utter cessation of the usual flow of ideas by association—to tranquillity within.

On Wholeness

Lat Pulldown

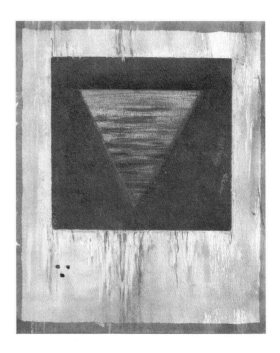

The mistake which many physical culturists make is . . . dividing the body into fragments with their "Knees Bend!" "Trunk Forward Bend!" "Eyes Right!" "Touch the Toes!" and so on. When I have asked you to turn your attention to a special part, it was with the object of exploring it, and not of exercising it as a thing separate from the rest of you.

—LOUISE MORGAN, *INSIDE YOURSELF*

The latissimus dorsi, the broad midback muscle, originates on the spinous processes (the bones you feel when you run your hand down the middle of your back) of the lower six thoracic vertebrae and all of the lumbar vertebrae, the lower three ribs, the back of the sacrum, and the posterior crests of the ilia (the ilia are the widest, uppermost, and largest sections of the pelvis). The lats insert near the top of the front of the humeri (upper arms). When displayed by a competitive bodybuilder, the great width of the lats resembles spread wings. Prominently developed lats form the upper portion of the "V" shape, an extensive upper-back tapering from the sides to a small waistline.

Their great length and breadth are what give the lats their powerful pulling action on the arms, enabling us to fully raise ourselves up by the arms. Which is why having strong lats appeals to our fantasies of adventure, especially rescue and escape from danger: dangling on a ledge high above the ground, we would use these mighty muscles to hoist ourselves up to safety. Down-to-earth, we weight-resistance yogins don't wish to sprout wings or have heroic strength. We just want to develop sufficient strength for everyday pulling activities.

But during the time we actually spend on strengthening the lats and other muscles, there's no concern for the consequences of our actions—not even for their beneficial effect on fitness. Throughout our busy day, we must constantly attend to actions that have consequences for us and for those for whom we're responsible; during the weight-resistance yoga session, however, we withdraw from the demands of quotidian reality to turn inward.

This inward stage begins with *ekagrata*, the one-point focus of dharana, concentration, the sixth of the eight limbs of classical hatha yoga. Unlike ordinary concentration, dharana is prolonged fixation on something—a fixation achieved by obliterating the ordinary means of perception and emptying the mind for the purpose of comprehending realities behind everyday life.

Following the yoga master B. K. S. Iyengar, who has shown how all eight limbs of classical hatha yoga are manifested in asana, weight-resistance yogins use our embodied experience of strengthening exercises as a vehicle for dharana. Our modern understanding of kinesiology and biomechanics has given us a detailed understanding of how movement against (and with) resistance works, enabling us to concentrate on the demands of the exercises at a far higher level than previously. Take, for example, the lat pulldown, one of the common exercises for the lats.

The lat pulldown is a relatively simple exercise: it basically consists of pulling an elevated bar down to the chest and returning the bar to the original position. Yet there's much to attend to. Consider just the moving parts involved in the pulling phase: the forearms bending at the elbows, the upper arms moving closer to the sides and somewhat back, and the shoulder blades brought back and down toward the spine. To ensure that these parts work efficiently, they must be moved moderately slowly in a precise range of motion. (In other words, no yanking.) To make these parts move forcefully, deliberately, smoothly, and securely demands the coordination of muscles of the upper limbs and trunk that generate, assist, guide, control, and stabilize the movements.

Ordinarily, weight lifters focus exclusively (but not often mindfully) on the parts of the body resisting the weights; but weight-resistance yogins also focus on those parts of the body not involved in the movement. Before we begin the lat pulldown proper, we fuss over the "inconsequential" parts (usually on the edges of, or not even in, the field of awareness of most weight lifters) to make them aligned and relaxed. The feet, a bit pigeon-toed, are firmly planted on the floor. The legs are squared, with the upper legs parallel to the floor and the lower legs perpendicular to the floor. The haunches (which include not only the buttocks but the upper thighs) are pulled back to accept the weight of the trunk. The spine is straightened, while retaining its natural curves (there's no exaggerated arch in the lumbar spine). The head is lined up with the spine, not bent back. Only after attaining this poised stillness—and while retaining concentration on these unmoving parts—do weight-resistance yogins then extend concentration to the moving parts.

This widening of attention to all parts of the body is what Iyengar identifies as dhyana, meditation, the seventh limb of hatha yoga. "Dharana is concentration on a point. Dhyana is concentration from that point without losing the source: 'Can I attend to the rest of the body?'"[2] However, dhyana is more than attention to an accumulation of parts. Through dhyana, we perceive the body in its wholeness.

"Can I extend my awareness of my self and bring it to each and every part of my body without any variation?" Iyengar asks, modeling the thinking process that takes place to make the transition from dharana to dhyana. "This is what I mean by fullness in meditation. I am full in my body."[3] Karl Baier, the philosopher of embodied yoga, describes the shift like this: "Then Asana becomes a way of being ourselves: No more 'I am turning my knee to the right' but 'I am entirely in the pose.'"[4] In bringing awareness from the separate parts of the body to the entire body during a weight-resistance yoga exercise, we expand our self and, in so doing, discover our self as embodied being.

When we perform with an awareness of the body in its entirety, our body becomes radiant. The moment we lose that full attention, our body becomes splintered, heavy, and dull. With an awareness of the body as a whole, we have a deep sense of our bodily existence, of dwelling within our body, of being at home in the world.

On Gravity

Shoulder Press

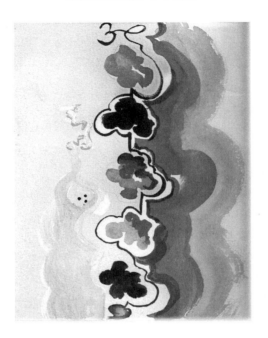

The movable object . . . adds on to its previous equable and indelible motion that downward tendency which it has from its own heaviness.

—GALILEO GALILEI, *TWO NEW SCIENCES*

Atlas led his fellow Titans in a losing battle against Zeus, the king of the gods. As punishment, Zeus forced Atlas to support the heavens on his shoulders forever. Curiously, many works of art show Atlas bearing the weight of Earth instead. Perhaps this is because we mortals so often feel the burden of "carrying the world on our shoulders."

Atlas was made to stand in the northwest region of what is now Africa, where the Atlas Mountains were named for him. Many weight lifters, perhaps intuitively emulating Atlas, stand like a mountain when performing the shoulder press. The risk in lifting a heavy weight directly above the shoulders in this unsupported position lies in the tendency to use the lower back, an area that should be stabilized, to help thrust up the weight, causing lower back strain.

Using a shoulder press machine focuses the contraction on the prime movers—the anterior, middle, and posterior fibers of the deltoid muscle—by restricting unnecessary joint movement and stabilizing the body. As is generally the case, performing the exercise with a machine is safer than with free weights.

Yet what makes free-weight exercises dangerous—their dependence on muscular coordination—is also what makes them advantageous. By involving stabilizing and guiding muscles to maintain control, free-weight exercises incorporate the use of more muscles and more closely mimic the required movements of everyday tasks. Free-weight exercises are only truly dangerous when they're practiced without strict attention to correct form. The considerable stress placed on the lower back by the unsupported shoulder press can be avoided by strongly co-contracting the lower back and abdominal muscles (or by reducing the weight or by simply sitting on a multi-angle bench adjusted to a slight incline) to keep the trunk stable.

Because free-weight exercises make use of gravity and not mechanical resistance, they are used to best effect when they optimally oppose gravity. Gravity, unlike the wind and other forces encountered by the body, behaves consistently and predictably; we have only to adapt to it by orientating ourselves in space. To optimally oppose gravity, we have to adjust our body (often with the aid of benches) to create a trajectory for our arms that requires shoulder, upper back, and chest muscles to overcome the greatest resistive force. (The path may put the weight load parallel to gravity, for example, in the front arm raise; diagonal to gravity, for example, in the shoulder diagonal raise; or perpendicular to gravity, for example, in the incline bench press.) As a consequence, during the course of performing a free-weight, upper-body exercise routine, which may comprise a dozen or so exercises, we find ourselves constantly repositioning our body and moving our arms at various angles. It's these alert, direct encounters with resisting the pull toward Earth's center that provide us with a unique opportunity to reflect on gravity.

By reflection on gravity I don't mean the study of gravity or even the mulling over of the essence of gravity but rather an opening up to gravity, an awareness of how gravity affects us. Performing the shoulder press may be only a hint, I admit, of the awareness of gravity that we would have in a rocket ship during lift off when the gravitational force to which our body is subjected is so great that it presses against our face, making it rubbery, or in an earthquake, when the ground before us suddenly opens up, hurling us down into a quarter mile-long crevasse. Nevertheless, while performing free-weight strengthening exercises we weight-resistance yogins have a keen sense of gravity on Earth. Especially during the shoulder press. In no other exercise do we resist gravity so clearly and mightily.

We could, of course, contemplate the effects of gravity during any activity—say, setting plates down on a table or putting the plates back in a cupboard. When we're going about our daily tasks, though, we can't allow ourselves to be bothered by thoughts about gravity. There's too much to get done. Unlike daily activities, which merely happen to involve gravity, lifting weights in the gymnasium lends itself to reflection on gravity, not only because it demands attentiveness to gravity and great effort against gravity but also because it's stripped of all everyday utility.

We could also go through our lives taking our movements with and against gravity for granted. But we shouldn't, for to pay attention to and control our interactions with gravity—just as with our breathing—is to begin to reflect on our very existence.

All objects attract each other with a force that's directly proportional to their masses. This law of gravity, discovered by Isaac Newton, applies to any object with mass (and, as was subsequently discovered, even to light), whether on Earth or in space. Because the force of Earth's gravitational attraction on the objects in its sphere is so much greater than the force of the objects (put simply, the objects are simply outweighed), we observe gravity as the force of Earth pulling objects down toward its center.

With the startling discovery of the universality of gravitation, we came to realize that seemingly unrelated things on and near Earth are alike. The moon spinning across the heavens. (If it weren't for its great velocity, the moon, like an iron ball shot out of a cannon, would eventually fall to Earth.) An apple falling from a tree to the ground. (For that matter, an apple lying on the ground. The force of gravity even acts on stationary objects resting on Earth's surface.) An atom. (If you dropped an atom, it would fall to the ground, just like an apple.) They're all affected by gravity—in this case, the great pull of Earth on objects within its sphere. (And what is Earth, after all, but a collection of atoms acting together to create one immense pull?)

Needless to say, human beings are subject to Earth's gravity, too. We continually oppose or surrender to gravity throughout our lives—for example, when lifting a heavy load and when lying down, respectively. In fact, we not only interact with gravity but have been formed by gravity. As a member of a species that evolved from water to land, we had to develop systems of structural support and locomotion that could adapt and even thrive in a terrestrial environment characterized, in part, by the resistance of its surface.

Insofar as we adjust in some way to Earth's gravity, we humans are brethren with all living things. For that matter, by being subject to Earth's gravity, we are like all things in Earth's sphere, inorganic as well as organic. We all have weight. We're all pulled down. We're all part of what in yoga is called *tamas*, inertia, heaviness, or sluggishness—one of the three *gunas* (the other two are *rajas*, motion, energetic action, or restlessness, and *sattwa*, moderation, orderliness, or harmony). These three qualities compose *prakriti*, the ordinary material world (reality manifested to the senses). We're all a part of this primordial matter. It's creation itself. In yoga it's commonly referred to as the Divine Mother, the avatar of prakriti. We're all born from the Divine Mother, and we all return to the Divine Mother.

On Right Tension

Seated Low Row

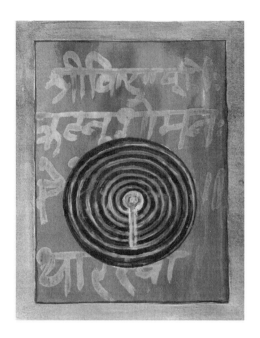

It is characteristic of our time that people look only for ways and means of achieving right relaxation without giving much thought to what is right tension.

—Karlfried Graf Von Dürckheim, *Hara*

The seated low row is one of the most inviting exercises in the gym, because it mirrors rowing a boat—for most of us, a seemingly pleasurable long-ago pastime. While performing the exercise, we can imagine ourselves, like the rowers in an Eakins painting, in the heat of competition, fiercely propelling a single-scull down the flat waters of the Schuylkill River. By turns, we mightily pull back on the oars and let ourselves be pulled forward—rhythmic motions against and with the water.

By lurching back and quickly releasing our trunk, we alternately recruit as many muscles as possible and save energy. Which is exactly why these movements are efficient for rowing—but inefficient, at best, and injurious, at worst, for strength training.

Some may not even realize that the seated low row, often performed by pulling back on a handle attached by a cord to a weight stack, is a shoulder joint extension exercise that primarily calls on back muscles to do the work. The muscles most involved are the latissimus dorsi and teres major, as well as the lower fibers of the pectoralis major—all of which cross the shoulder joint to insert on the upper arm.

Targeting these muscles is made inefficient—not to mention unsafe—when we lunge back with our lower back and push off with our legs to help pull the weights up, and then let the hasty descent of the weights jerk us forward, greatly relieved at having a couple of seconds of rest before starting over. By involving irrelevant muscles, using momentum, and allowing limpness, we impede the muscles most involved, keeping them from fully doing their work.

The correct form for the seated low row is relatively easy to learn. The back is kept upright. The legs are kept still. The initial (positive) movement is performed at a moderately slow speed, with control, which allows the targeted muscles to apply near maximum force and maintain tension. Although involving great effort, this pulling movement can be said to be carried out without strain because it not only springs forth from a relaxed, yet alert, stillness but also is performed with care.

During the return (negative) movement, the shoulder blades are moved in a restrained manner, as if we're honoring their reluctance to go to the aid of the overbearing arms. The arms aren't allowed to go slack; they're released in a slow, controlled manner. By only gradually giving in to the pull of the weights during this final movement, we strengthen the latissimus dorsi and other muscles yet again, this time while they're elongating. Because the muscles most involved remain taut, this letting go movement can be said to be carried out with effort.

Yet even after we've learned how to correct the wasteful and reckless rowing movements, we still find it hard to give them up. They enable us to pull a heavier load. They can be performed wholeheartedly. All in all, they feel comfortable—absolutely normal—while the correct movements feel diminished and unnatural. So why change? But when practicing weight-resistance yoga, which is steeped in the yogic refusal to conform to our most basic inclinations, stopping to rethink and change our habitual movements is exactly what we do.

■

The issue, however, goes beyond efficiency and even avoidance of injury. How we deal with tension and release in strength training is an indication of how we conduct our life. In our swing from clumsily lurching back to passively jerking forward, we're making our private life public. There in the gym, it's as if we're beginning sex with much awkward flailing, and then it's quickly over with. Or we're agitated at the office, only to fall into a TV-watching stupor at home. Or we're irritable one day (*better stay away from me*), then sentimental and lugubrious the next. Or we're an anxious careerist for most of our lives, then find ourselves a bored retiree. The rhythm of our intimate moments, the pattern of our days, our very fate is exposed in our motions.

In weight-resistance yoga, we put an end to the cycle of yanking or shoving weights followed by letting them fly or drop back. Instead, we perform both the weight bearing and the letting go with the right tension. With the result that effort in movement and relaxation in movement become nearly the same. In so doing, we find a model for dealing with tension and release in a way that may carry over to and improve our everyday life. And, more importantly, we allow for transcending our everyday life during the session.

During each session the weight-resistance yogin suspends the human condition, which is characterized, in part, by the necessity to recognize dualities. For example, those dualities we teach our children to help them adapt to the world: sense of self and sense of others; overregulated impulses and uncontrolled impulses; wishes and reality-orientated thinking. In moving deliberatively with relaxed tension and tense release, accompanied by rhythmic breathing, we yogins transcend the dualities of tension and release. This unity of effort and relaxation (it perhaps still needs to be said) isn't symbolic—or rather, isn't only symbolic. We experience it within our own body.

Romanian yoga scholar Mircea Eliade describes the primordial unity as "the undifferentiated completeness of precreation."[5] This unity was separated into dualities in order to form the stuff of everyday life. Through the *act* of reuniting the dualities of tension and release within our own body, we open up the possibility of reuniting all of the polar principles—but most pointedly, immobility and mobility, self and world, death and life, nonbeing and Being.

On Harmony

Standing High Row

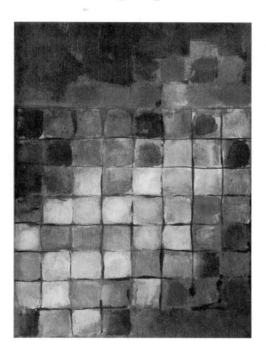

Maybe you have read the Bhagavad Gita, where we are asked
to keep the body in a rhythmic, harmonious state without any
variations between the right and the left, the front and the back,
measuring from the central line of the body which runs from the
middle of the throat to the middle of the anus.

—B. K. S. Iyengar, *The Tree of Yoga*

You can spot musclebound weight lifters without even seeing their massive chests and rounded shoulders. As they trundle away from you on the gym floor, a small telltale sign betrays them: their hands facing you. This cartoonish trait results from overdeveloping the chest muscles to the point where they pull on the shoulders, causing the arms to rotate inward, which twists the hands around until the palms face back. (In his desire to display his virility, a friend's teenage son, who very recently started lifting weights at a gym, has begun to ape this mannerism of maladaptation and the accompanying lumbering gait—even at home, where nobody is impressed.)

In contrast to the pectoralis major (the thick, fan-shaped muscle that makes up the bulk of the chest muscles), the infraspinatus is decidedly not a glamour muscle. Only part of it can be seen (on the upper back below the posterior deltoid and the spine of the shoulder blade), and it isn't very big. Because it's not much to show off, weight lifters tend to ignore it. It is, however, the largest of the rotator cuff muscles—those muscles originating on the shoulder blade that provide stability to the humeral socket by interweaving over the shoulder joint capsule and inserting on the head of the upper arm. Alone among the rotator cuff muscles, though, the infraspinatus has another critical function: along with the teres minor and posterior and middle fibers of the deltoid, it pulls the shoulders back, thereby strengthening the upper back and opening up the chest.

The choreography of the weight-resistance exercise routine is determined by several factors. Upper-body joint movements are worked one day, lower-body joint movements, the next day. Exercises increase in difficulty at the beginning of a routine and decrease in difficulty at the end of a routine. Each series of exercises revolves around a different joint. Exercises within a series may complete a range of motion or may work slightly different planes of motion. But no organizing principles are more important to the weight-resistance yoga exercise routine than balance (pairing opposing muscles) and symmetry (pairing left and right muscles).

Which is why all of us who perform an exercise that moves the upper arm in the horizontal plane toward the chest (to strengthen the pectoralis major), such as the chest press, should also perform an exercise that moves the upper arm in the horizontal plane away from the chest (to strengthen the infraspinatus), such as the high row. These two shoulder joint exercises—one pushing and one pulling—when paired together, are called opposing, contralateral, or balancing exercises (analogous to weight-surrender yoga's neutralizing or counter poses).

And which is why if we perform a high row for the right side, we should perform a high row for the left side. In performing symmetrical exercises, we establish on either side of the spine (the left/right dividing line of the body) similarity of arrangement—a correspondence not only of right and left muscles in size and shape, but also, more importantly, of right and left bones in aligned positions.

Around 1490 Leonardo da Vinci completed his famous pen-and-ink drawing of the naked, curly-headed, tender-looking figure with perfect proportions named *Vitruvian Man*. *Vitruvian Man*'s perfection is demonstrated by his ability to fit his body to the perfect geometric forms—a circle and a square—by opening his legs and raising his outstretched arms in a kind of jumping jack. In this image, in which a naturalistically rendered man incongruously stands on and touches a circle and square that enclose him, the perfect proportions of the human body become an analogy for the harmony, the ordered whole, of the cosmos.

In practicing weight-resistance yoga, we don't achieve perfect head, limb, and trunk proportions. (Of course, there's no such thing as a universal set of proportions for the human body. Rarely is a man's height exactly the length of twenty-four palms or are his outspread arms exactly equal to his height. We all have individual variations. In any case, there's nothing we can do to change our proportions.) Still, by performing strengthening exercises for the front and back, left and right, upper and lower, and exterior and interior of the body, we forge a body that's balanced and symmetrical—a body configured to the harmony of its own unique skeletal structure. Possessing a musculature that harmoniously arranges our skeletal structure allows us to sit or stand in comfortable and effortless positions. When muscles properly align bones, the strain, fatigue, and weakness caused by habitually faulty alignment (what we commonly call poor posture) are eliminated.

David Gordon White, scholar of the alchemical body, argues against the interpretation of yoga as solely "a meditative practice through which the absolute [is] to be found by turning the mind and senses inward, away from the world."[6] In opposition to this closed model, he asserts, there's a yoga tradition of an open model of the human body—a model that links the body and the cosmos. But these two models aren't dichotomous. As yoga scholar Mircea Eliade argues: "In withdrawing from profane human life, the yogin finds another that is deeper and truer—the very life of the cosmos."[7] Thusly, taking a static bodily position, breathing rhythmically, closing off the distractions of sensory activity, concentrating on a single point, and fixing the flux of consciousness are explained "by the intention to homologize the body and life of man with the celestial bodies and cosmic rhythms, first of all with the sun and moon."[8]

In having the sensation (produced by coupling weight-resistance yoga upper- and lower-body workouts) of our major bones precisely fitting together and our major muscles being superbly toned and relaxed, we experience direct knowledge of the harmony within our own body. Through contemplation of this bodily harmony—which is to say, the essence of our body—we experience (it's impossible to prevent!) a correspondence with the harmony of the cosmos, accompanied by a great calm.

MEDITATIONS ON THE ELBOW JOINT

■ **On Enchanted Space—Introduction to the Elbow Joint**

I think of dumbbells and barbells as hand tools. Admittedly, they're peculiar hand tools. Used for lifting and lowering exercises, they don't save energy or produce great force. To the contrary: using them commonly expends more energy than carrying out daily activities with similar movements.

■ **On Energy—Standing Biceps Curl and Triceps Pushdown**

Some women consider arms an accoutrement to fashion; they diligently work their triceps at the gym so they can expose tanned, toned arms in summer dresses. Some men display sixteen-inch biceps in T-shirts and tank tops as a sign of their virility. But this fetishizing of arms shouldn't turn us off to the beauty of arms with subtle definition. Even in the streets of New York City, those women and men who take a stroll on a sunny summer afternoon with bared, toned arms swinging freely and jauntily from their shoulders attain at least a hint of the grace of leopards, snakes, giraffes, and other wild animals of the jungle.

On Enchanted Space

Introduction to the Elbow Joint

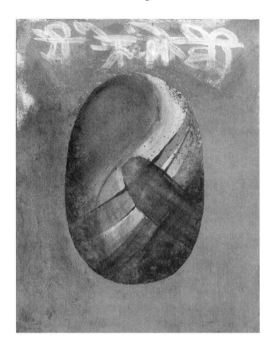

*One should become void in and void out, like a pot in cosmic
space. Full within and full without, like a jar in the ocean.*

—Svatmarama, *The Hatha Yoga Pradipika*

I think of dumbbells and barbells as hand tools. Hand tools are used for performing manual work on some sort of material. We use them to knock, chop, cut,
smooth, drill, measure, level, grip, pry open, twist, hold, raise, grind, and dig up
the material. Using hand tools such as pliers or a mallet saves energy because these
tools, in effect, amplify the force of our muscles in carrying out tasks. Some tasks,
like dislodging a large rock, would be impossible to perform without having a
hand tool (in this case, a crowbar) to increase the force exerted. As our ancestors
discovered about 2.6 million years ago when they used sharpened stones for hunt-
ing, hand tools are efficient and powerful extensions of our bodies.

Admittedly, dumbbells and barbells are peculiar hand tools. Used for lifting and
lowering exercises, they don't save energy or produce great force. To the contrary:

using them commonly expends more energy than carrying out daily activities with similar movements. Moreover, the material to which these tools are applied is, of all things, the very one that's used to initiate the force: our muscles.

Bend your elbow, and release it. Then take hold of a dumbbell. Bend your elbow again. Because the resistance to flexing your elbow joint increases, the muscle force must also increase. And that's the point. By gradually adding resistance during strength training, we find the optimal overload needed for the most efficient strength gain. In contrast to, say, hitting a nail with a hammer, or, for that matter, hitting a baseball with a bat (activities which are directed toward the world), lifting weights to transform our muscles (by making them bigger and stronger) is self-referential—and risks being self-centered.

The most powerful muscles that operate the hand at the wrist originate on the upper arm and cross the forearm as well as the wrist. (A power grip—the whole hand wrapped around something—significantly relies on these relatively strong wrist joint muscles. This is easily illustrated by grasping a hammer: you can instantly see—and feel—how the muscles on your forearm tighten up in isometric contraction.) But most hand-tool use involves the coordination of wrist, forearm, elbow, shoulder, and even torso movements. In hand-tool movements in which the wrists are kept straight (as they generally should be to make the hands less vulnerable to injury), the movements are almost solely controlled by muscles that bend the elbow (the biceps brachii, the brachialis, and the brachioradialis) and straighten the elbow (the triceps brachii). (This is also illustrated by using a hammer: if you're not simply tapping it, elbow movements are forcefully brought into play.) If the forearm twists during the movement, the muscles that rotate the forearm externally (biceps brachii and brachioradialis) and/or internally (brachioradialis) are involved.

Considering that elbow and forearm joint muscles are used to strengthen the muscles that manipulate tools, it's hardly surprising that elbow and forearm joint exercises resemble dipping a ladle into a pot, pulling on a fishing line, turning a screwdriver, and the like. In fact, one of advantages of dumbbells and barbells (as well as free motion machines and as opposed to variable-resistance machines) is that using them requires a pattern of intra- and intermuscular coordination that more closely mimics the movement requirements of everyday tasks—including tool use.

"The thoughtful maker of cabinets," observes the philosopher David Michael Levin, ". . . takes pride in his tools, and handles them with a timeless care. As he planes the wood, he caresses the grain. In the flow of his movements we will observe poise and grace; and in his gentle touching and holding we may sense a visible tact."[1] We weight-resistance yogins, artisans of sorts, express our reverence for our tools—dumbbells and barbells—by using them with the same grace, consideration, and care. Dumbbells are cautiously picked up from the rack, as are plates from the weight tree. During an exercise, dumbbells aren't clanged together. After an exercise, they aren't abruptly dropped to the floor. Dumbbells are returned to the racks, and plates to the weight trees, with the care of an antique dealer setting down an ancient vase. (This reverence also applies to those amazing contraptions, weight-resistance machines.)

When we become deeply in touch with the value of our tools, we find ourselves going about our exercises free of ego-attachments and aversions (you know what I mean: fantasies, regrets, doubts, complaints, and such). Having an awareness of our tools is a means of thinking less about ourselves—which, it turns out, isn't so much a cultural prescription as a built-in biological mechanism.

An infant in the early stage of development (when language is just beginning to form) acquires knowledge about the world primarily by coordinating sensory experiences (such as seeing and hearing) with physical (motor) actions. Between four and eight months, the infant, moving beyond self-preoccupation (with his or her own body), becomes more object-oriented. Vision and prehension are coordinated. The infant intentionally grasps for a desired object.

While performing a weight-resistance yoga exercise routine, when dumbbells and barbells are handled with deliberation, this preverbal sensorimotor field opens up to us. It's not just that we comprehend what we ordinarily take for granted: that objects are separate from the self and permanent (in the sense that they exist when we're absent). Or even that we experience the inherent pleasure in grasping objects. It's that we have an awareness of the clearing within which these objects are revealed to us. And we have a wondrous sense of the unbounded expanse that surrounds these man-made objects—the immensities of sea and land. In this way, the world around us is transformed. We find ourselves, in Levin's description, in "a space of enchantment."[2]

On Energy
Standing Biceps Curl and Triceps Pushdown

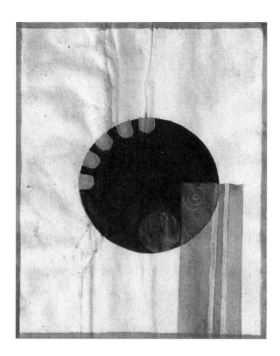

By meditating on anything as oneself, man becomes that.

—GANDHARVA TANTRA

*Of what is and has been and is to be, and what moves or remains
still, the sun alone is the source and the end.*

—ATTRIBUTED TO SAUNAKA, *BRHAD-DEVATA*

Some women consider arms an accoutrement to fashion. Disgusted by the jiggly
flesh of flabby underarms, they diligently work their triceps at the gym so they
can expose tanned, toned arms in summer dresses. Some men display sixteen-
inch biceps in T-shirts and tank tops as a sign of their virility. (Some wags say
that men want strong biceps to pull women toward them, and that women want
strong triceps to push men away.) But this fetishizing of arms shouldn't turn us
off to the beauty of arms with subtle definition. Even in the streets of New York
City, those women and men who take a stroll on a sunny summer afternoon

with bared, toned arms swinging freely and jauntily from their shoulders attain at least a hint of the grace of leopards, snakes, giraffes, and other wild animals of the jungle. All the more reason to be surprised (and perhaps deflated) upon realizing how utterly mechanically our arms work.

Like most of the levers in the human body, the elbow joint is a third-class lever, classified as such because the force to move a bony part is applied between the axis and the resistance. Specifically, the force of the biceps muscles (which originate on the front of the shoulder and arm) to bend the forearm is applied at an insertion on the top of the forearm just *below* the elbow joint—so the insertion is between the axis (the elbow joint) and the resistance (in the middle of the top of the forearm).

But the elbow joint is also a first-class lever, classified as such because the force to move a bony part is applied on the side of the axis away from the resistance. Specifically, the force of the triceps muscles (which originate on the back of the shoulder and arm) to straighten the forearm is applied at an insertion on the bottom of the forearm just *above* the elbow joint—so the axis (the elbow joint) is between the insertion and the resistance (in the middle of the bottom of the forearm). Thus the elbow joint (when bending) is not so different, really, from a screen door operated by a short spring, but the elbow joint (when straightening) is not so different from a seesaw, either.

In the human body, these kinds of levers permit a wide range of motion in only one plane. The three elbow flexors (biceps brachii, brachialis, and brachioradialis) primarily bring the forearm toward the shoulder by bending the elbow. The three heads of triceps brachii primarily take the forearm away from the shoulder by straightening the elbow.

Although a muscle is a mechanical device, its energy to move parts of the body is produced by a chemical reaction: changes in the configuration of the muscle on a molecular level. In dramatic contrast to the electric motor or turbojet, muscle depends on what might be called a molecular engine (a soft, wet, and contractile engine, but an engine nevertheless). As Steven Vogel, historian of muscle, observes, "Cross-bridges between protein molecules are fabulously tiny engines . . . harnessed in long and broad arrays [to] produce large-scale, forceful motion."[3] This was essentially proven about seventy years ago.

In 1938 in Hungary, the acclaimed physiologist Albert Szent-Györgyi (who had received the Nobel Prize for discovering vitamin C) began research on how skeletal muscle fibers accomplish their mechanical work. In 1940, he extracted the muscle protein myosin from rabbit muscle, drew it into a hypodermic syringe, and then spurted it into a solution, forming fine threads. When he added adenosine triphosphate (ATP), a complex chemical compound found in muscles that releases a great amount of energy (extracted from nutrients—that is, food that's eaten) when its phosphate bonds are split, the threads rapidly contracted to one-third their original size, mimicking muscle fiber tensing. Chemical energy had been converted into mechanical work! (Szent-Györgyi and his team subsequently showed how myosin combines with another muscle protein, actin, to contract muscle when ATP releases energy. So it's actually through the formation of actomyosin that muscle produces force, creating the body's ability to do work.)

Szent-Györgyi later commented that, upon seeing the myosin contract in his original experiments, he was observing "one of the oldest and most mysterious signs of life—motion—reproduced for the first time in vitro."[4] If movement helps define animal life and muscle enables movement, then muscle, Szent-Györgyi demonstrated, is essential to animal life.

Part of the luminous energy of the sun pours down on Earth. Although some of this light is reflected, most is absorbed. "On this day, and the next day, and every day," science writer Oliver Morton observes, the sun's "scarcely conceivable" energy warms the sky and "the land and the sea, its warmth driving the winds and ocean currents."[5] A tiny amount of this solar energy is absorbed not by inanimate objects but by plants that transform it, by photosynthesis, into chemical energy. Through Earth's food web, this energy is transferred from organism to organism: plants grow, animals eat plants, and animals eat animals.

For this reason, if there were no sun, there wouldn't be any animal life—which includes, of course, any human life. The sun's energy, transmuted, flows through us as it has flowed through almost all of Earth's life for at least 3.8 billion years. (As Morton points out, Earth is hardly a lonely planet.) While performing a weight-resistance yoga exercise routine, we comprehend in our very sinews that the sun makes life possible on Earth; that the mechanical work of muscles—motion—is ultimately generated by solar energy; that, therefore, each movement we take partakes of a cosmological dimension.

As a consequence of this comprehension, during the weight-resistance yoga session—which becomes a kind of rite—we weight-resistance yogins discard our usual identities (formed by work, family, religion, gender, age, creed, race, community, or country) and, instead, define ourselves as followers of Surya, the sun god, the heavenly fire that illumines the world. Not followers in the crude sense that we worship or pray to Surya but in the sense that we recognize, as yoga scholar Alain Daniélou elucidates in his book on the gods of India, that Surya and other deities are "the manifestations of distinct powers springing from an unknowable 'Immensity.'"[6]

In attaining experiential knowledge of movement—one of the essential elements of animal life—we find ourselves oriented to the sun. Through our bodily communion with this heavenly shining body twirling distantly in space, the intimacy of our human solitude blends with the Immensity.

MEDITATIONS
ON THE SHOULDER GIRDLE

■ **On Fragility—Introduction to the Shoulder Girdle**

Weight-resistance yogins commonly concentrate on the movement of joints—movements generally allowed by the subtle interplay of groups of muscles. We marvel at a mobile joint's "opening," and "closing." But weight-resistance yoga is defined just as much by restraint of movement as by movement. So we also sometimes concentrate on the stability of joints—stability maintained by strong tissues that allow little or no motion. We find that a secure joint, while mechanically explicable, contains just as much a mystery as a joint that freely moves.

■ **On the Silent Sound—Shoulder Pulldown and Shoulder Shrug**

When Darwin was doing research for *The Expression of Emotions in Man and Animals,* he sent questionnaires to missionaries around the world to find out if any gestures familiar to people in the West existed in other cultures. What he learned was that shrugging the shoulders is not only the single gesture common to all peoples but is also innate. We all, Darwin discovered, shrug our shoulders to show our helplessness and impotence. But for weight-resistance yoga practitioners, the shrugging movement isn't a form of communication: it's simply an exercise for strengthening the middle fibers of the trapezius.

On Fragility

Introduction to the Shoulder Girdle

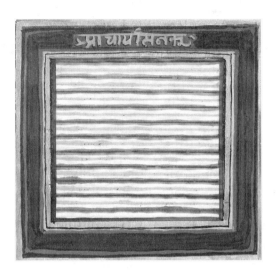

*[When St. Francis stood on his head,] he might see and love every
tile on the steep roofs or every bird on the battlements; but he
would see them all in a new and divine light of eternal danger
and dependence. Instead of being merely proud of his strong city
because it could not be moved, he would be thankful to God
Almighty that it had not been dropped. . . .*

—G. K. CHESTERTON, *ST. FRANCIS OF ASSISI*

What chatterboxes we are—even in solitude! Yogins seek to stop this psychomental flux by fixing our mind on a single point. Fixing our mind is a prerequisite for experiencing comprehensions of reality. What we fix our mind on
determines what aspect of reality we comprehend.

Nothing if not practical and concrete, yogic philosophy suggests several possible aids for fixing the mind, such as having a mental image of a Lord, chanting a
mantra, or staring at burning coals or a *mandala*. For those of us involved in the
embodied practices of weight-surrender or weight-resistance yoga, concentrating on
a part of the body as the single point at which to fix our attention is particularly apt.

Traditionally in yoga, the parts of the body concentrated on are the navel,
the lotus of the heart (the solar plexus), the forehead, the tip of the nose, the

tip of the tongue, or the area between the eyes. These locations, however, hold no meaning for those of us who perform yogic stretching and strengthening: they're arbitrary and ideological. As an alternative, we find locations that are relevant to our embodied practices as we experience them.

These holy places to which we, like pilgrims, make a journey include the crown of the head, nape of the neck, armpits, crooks of the elbows, pit of the stomach, linea alba (the line that separates the left and right rectus abdominis muscles), small of the back, sacrum, pubic symphysis (where the left and right pubic bones meet), knobby sitting bones, perineum (the area between the anus and the genitals), hollows of the knees, heels of the feet, and other locations of the bodily landscape.

Some of these places are joints. Weight-resistance yogins commonly concentrate on the movement of joints, such as back and forth and side to side—movements generally allowed by the subtle interplay of groups of muscles. We marvel at a mobile joint's "opening," and "closing." But weight-resistance yoga is defined just as much by restraint of movement as by movement. So we also sometimes concentrate on the stability of joints—stability maintained by strong tissues that allow little or no motion. We find that a secure joint, while mechanically explicable, contains just as much a mystery as a joint that freely moves.

Although the shoulder girdle—the shoulder blades (scapulae) and collar bones (clavicles)—sits on the trunk like a harness, reminding us that we're beasts of burden (this bony structure, is, after all, essential to carrying buckets of water and pulling wagons), the shoulder girdle movements themselves are small (mere twitches, really, especially compared to extravagant upper-limb movements) and, on the whole, not conducive to labor. Common examples of shoulder girdle movement are squinching the right and left halves of the upper back together to alleviate back strain, pulling the shoulders down in a well-executed *Bhujangasana,* Cobra Pose, shrugging in incomprehension, and shimmying on the dance floor. These movements are carried out by the trapezius, levator scapulae, rhomboids, serratus anterior, and pectoralis minor muscles.

The spatial relationships of the movement of these muscles are defined in terms of their positions to the shoulder blades (e.g., shoulder girdle adduction, or retraction, produced by contraction of the rhomboids, is the pulling back of the shoulder blades towards the spine). However, the sternoclavicular joint—the place where the small heads of the collarbones attach to the sternum (the flat, dagger-shaped breastplate)—is where the essence of the shoulder girdle is comprehended. The shoulder blades participate in every upper-arm movement and may move in a variety of directions on their own. But it's the tiny articulations of the collarbones with the sternum that provide the only bony link of the shoulder girdle (and therefore of the arms, which dangle from the shoulder blades) to the trunk.

Only about 50 percent of the heads of the collarbones attach at the fossae (small depressions) of the manubrium, the broad, top segment of the sternum, leaving the shoulder girdle precariously balanced. Or so it would seem. In fact, there's a surprising strength and stability in this synovial joint: on every side, structural supports reinforce the joint, making dislocations uncommon. Yet, if some misfortune were to befall us, and a great force (a mallet brought down on a chisel!) were applied between the collarbones and the two shallow pits where the bones attach at the sternum, the entire, elaborate shoulder apparatus, including the arms, would separate from the axial skeleton (the skull, vertebral column, sternum, and ribs). And that's the point. We're ultimately drawn to this joint not for its stability but for its quality of fragility.

Seen in this light, fixing our attention (in our mind's eye) on the sternoclavicular joint—or, more sensibly, on the place just above where the collarbones meet, the small hollow into which we could press a thumb—while performing shoulder girdle exercises shakes our confidence. We know that our body could (inevitably will) collapse into a heap of bones. We're shaken in our assumptions of all solidity. Everything could change, we realize, in less time than it takes to sigh, as the result of a stumble on stairs; a minor automobile collision; the collapse of a skyscraper struck by airplanes; the rubbing of tectonic plates, which unleashes an earthquake; the wayward path of a comet; or cosmic overextension, causing the universe to implode. Our lifetime, Earth's history, the unfolding of the universe itself—all could come to an end.

Comprehending our precariousness, we're left with a sense of the holiness of the intricate structure of our muscles and bones. This bodily experience of stability opens us up to an awareness of infinite Being that holds and supports the earth and all life on it. For yogins, the embodiment of this phenomenon is Lord Ananta, the endless (and therefore eternal) snake who encircles Earth, holding it steadily in place on His hood. We perform our exercises in an aura of giving thanks to Him for our body being held together. We're filled with gratitude to Him that all things haven't yet fallen apart.

On the Silent Sound

Shoulder Pulldown and Shoulder Shrug

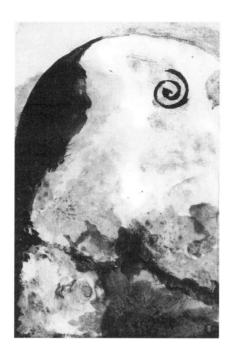

*The union of mind and the [unmade] sound is called Raja-Yoga.
. . . Those who are ignorant of the Raja-Yoga and practice only the
Hatha-Yoga, will, in my opinion, waste their energy fruitlessly.*

—Svatmarama, *Hatha Yoga Pradipika*

When Darwin was doing research for *The Expression of Emotions in Man and Animals* (1872), he sent questionnaires to missionaries around the world to find out if any gestures familiar to people in the West existed in other cultures. What he learned was that shrugging the shoulders—raising both shoulders with a quick movement—is not only the single gesture common to all peoples but is also innate. Whether young children or the blind, people of this race or people of that religion, Europeans or "natives having had scarcely any intercourse with Europeans,"[1] "the wild Indian tribes of the western parts of the United States,"[2] or "the hill-tribes of India,"[3] we all, Darwin discovered, shrug our shoulders, and for the same reason: to show our helplessness and impotence.

But for weight-resistance yoga practitioners, the shrugging movement isn't a form of communication: it's simply an exercise for strengthening the middle fibers of the trapezius, commonly called "the traps" (the pair of large, flat, triangular muscles on the upper back), to enable them to better elevate the shoulder blades. Although somewhat involved in various actions such as holding objects out to the side or high overhead, the middle traps, assisted by the weaker upper traps (which elevate the collarbones), are strenuously involved in pulling objects straight up with a shrugging movement, such as lifting the handles of a wheelbarrow.

The problem for many of us isn't so much that our middle and upper traps are weak but that they're habitually scrunched up. So why would we want to reinforce this tension by strengthening already tense muscles? The answer is, we wouldn't. We're better off stretching them ("Pull your shoulders away from your ears," our weight-surrender yoga instructor gently chides us during *Urdhva Mukha Svanasana,* Upward Facing Dog Pose) and strengthening the muscles that oppose them (by pulling down against resistance using the fibers of the lower traps). Once the middle and upper traps have attained a normal resting length, we can then set about strengthening them along with the lower traps.

In fact, no aspect of weight-resistance yoga is a form of communication. The weight-resistance yoga session is a form of tapas, or austerity, practiced in quiet and calm. Like an asana class, the strength-exercise yoga session is not only without music but also without conversation. Weight-resistance yogins never speak or allow themselves to be spoken to while performing an exercise. Not only speech but also gestures and facial expressions—which reveal our thoughts and feelings—are absent. To enter the gymnasium floor, the sacred space, is to take a vow of silence. During the session, we are *munis,* those who practice silence (abstention from speech).

During this time, when we're cut off from all social interaction, we may feel anxious and lonely (as we commonly do when practicing hatha yoga)—at least, at first. But the isolation enables us to become fully absorbed in our tasks, shutting out all that normally stimulates our senses and presenting us with the possibility of a breakthrough in sensory receptivity—a prerequisite for reaching samadhi (the comprehension of realities, hidden during everyday life, that can only take place when all concern with the self has been disregarded). First, I listen attentively to the ordinary sounds around me. Then, I listen for anahata nada—the sound that remains in the absence of all other sounds, the sound made without the contact of two objects, the unmade sound.

Most of the time we're too caught up in the hubbub of daily life not only to practice silence but to listen to silence. We're usually listening to voices (my wife asking me to add milk to the shopping list) or music (the *Goldberg Variations* on the speaker system) or noises (a car backing out of a parking space at the shopping mall as we walk toward the supermarket entrance). Our ability to carry out ordinary tasks, our capacity for aesthetic pleasure, our very survival depend on our attention to such sounds.

However, there are times—such as walking on a path in the woods or lying in a post-coital embrace or falling off to sleep in the afternoon—when I find myself, through no effort of my own, listening to anahata nada. It's the outward sign that I'm perfectly happy.

The weight-resistance yoga session is a systematic effort to bring forth this sound, or, rather, to become aware of it. For anahata nada is always present. It must merely be brought into consciousness. Neither the inhibition of the senses of touch, sight, smell, and taste nor the total absence of voices, music, noise, and other sounds is enough to enable us to hear this sound. It requires a kind of attentiveness.

In my experience, anahata nada is often initially rather violent, like the rush of stormy ocean waves on the shore. Somewhat panicked, I want to flee from it. (There's very little in hatha yoga that doesn't have its unnerving and even frightening aspect.) After overcoming my anxiety, I find the sound gradually becoming more and more refined, until it's something like a thin musical hum. And then, whether or not I want it to happen, I find that my listening is accompanied by a great calm.

When we listen to anahata nada, we aren't deaf to other sounds in the world. It's not that other sounds are stopped or not heard. How can they be? It's just that they drop into this sound, like stones dropping into the middle of the ocean.

Anahata nada is the primordial sound, the sound before time, before sound was made by two objects. It's the same sound that our ancestors heard and that our descendants will hear. It's the universal sound, present everywhere. It's within us, and all around us. It is, you could say, the song of the soul and the cosmos.

MEDITATIONS ON THE TRUNK
(VERTEBRAL COLUMN AND ABDOMINAL WALL)

■ On Mortality—Introduction to the Trunk

Far more than any other bony part, the spinal column—the most complex part of the human body after the brain and central nervous system—seems to be the essence of the skeleton. In our mind's eye, the spine evokes the skeleton as a whole. Awareness of our spine comes especially to the fore during trunk exercises—back extensions, sit-ups, side twists, and side bends—in which the upper and lower limbs neither assist nor initiate movement.

■ On Nonviolence—Back Raise

The upward phase of the back raise, the strengthening exercise performed while lying face down on the Roman chair, resembles Bhujangasana, Cobra Pose. In this position, I think of myself not as a cobra in a dense highland forest but as a seahorse bobbing around in sea grass meadows, mangrove stands, or coral reefs.

■ On Withdrawal—Ab Curl

During deep, or forced, breathing, previously dormant muscles are recruited to meet the increased demands of expiration. The abdominal muscles play a critical role in forced expiration. When we consider the abdominals in light of this critical contribution to the process of deep breathing, we realize what ninnies we are to get caught up in wanting to sculpt a soft tummy into a tight, well-defined anterior abdominal wall for display.

On Mortality

Introduction to the Trunk

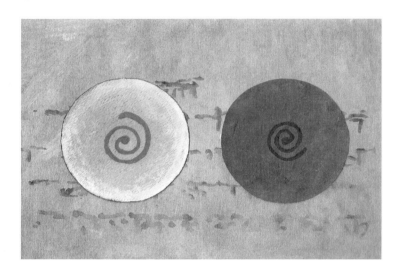

After quarreling with her wealthy husband, a beautiful young woman with a voluptuous figure, dressed in luxurious garments and adorned with ornaments, fled town in the early morning. Scurrying along the narrow dirt road to her family home, she bumped into a noble-looking young beggar, knocking him to the ground. When he looked up at her, she laughed flirtatiously, whether toying with him or genuinely trying to tempt him, we cannot say. As she hurried off, the beggar picked himself up and continued on his way.

A short while later, the plump husband, wearing a silk robe and slippers, running as fast as he could, appeared on the road. He rushed up to the beggar and, clearly beside himself, breathlessly asked, "Holy sir, have you seen a young woman who looks like a goddess pass this way?" The beggar replied, "Somebody passed by. Whether it was a man or a woman, I couldn't tell. What I saw was a skeleton, bones linked up with bones."

—BHADANTACARIYA BUDDHAGHOSA,
VISUDDHIMAGGA

We usually think of the vertebral column in terms of its contribution to upright posture. The cervical, thoracic, and lumbar vertebrae—the series of joined bones that form the movable spine (in our mind's eye, almost always pictured from the side)—must retain their natural curves for us to stand tall. From this sturdy column, aligned posture extends forward (to the ribs and sternum), upward (to the cranium), and downward (to the pelvis).

Connected to the spinal column in front are twelve pairs of ribs that form the greater part of the thorax (chest wall). The ten upper ribs are connected to the sternum (breastbone). Together, the twenty-six vertebrae, twenty-four ribs, and sternum make up the trunk. The spine supports the cranium (head). And the spine, in turn, is supported on the pelvis: the second to the last vertebra, the broad sacrum—the body's holy bone—is wedged between the pelvic bones like a keystone in a bridge.

Of course, bones don't support themselves. Activated muscles provide them with mechanical stability. And these same muscles that hold the trunk bones in place allow for their movements: bending the trunk forward, bending the trunk backward, twisting the trunk, and bending sideways. Muscles attached to the spine and pelvis (such as the large erector spinae in the back) and muscles attached to the ribs and pelvis (such as the large abdominal muscles in the front) not only provide trunk stability and movement but also protect the internal organs.

Far more than any other bony part, the vertebral column—the most complex part of the human body after the brain and central nervous system—seems to be the essence of the skeleton. In our mind's eye, the spine evokes the skeleton as a whole. Awareness of our spine comes especially to the fore during trunk exercises: back extensions, sit-ups, side twists, and side bends. Our appendages neither assist nor initiate movement during these exercises; knowing their place, the arms are either considerately folded across the chest or dutifully grasping weights, and the legs are responsibly secured.

By bringing awareness to our spine, trunk exercises evoke our evolutionary past—our gradual change through long eras of time from previously existing forms. They connect us to our vertebral ancestors—from apes, the fellow mammals from whom we've most recently evolved, back to reptiles, to amphibians, and ultimately to the earliest vertebrates, fish. Specifically, the primitive eel-like

Agnatha, a largely extinct class which declined some 380 million years ago but which includes two living groups, the blood-sucking lampreys and the scavenging hagfishes. (Even these earliest-known vertebrates had skeletons made up of bone, enamel, dentine, and cartilage—the four basic tissues that make up our skeletons.)

During trunk exercises, while some may feel that they're like rising and falling snakes on the ground, I have the sensation that I'm barely terrestrial at all, that I'm in the primeval aquatic element: the sea. Although we're remaining in place—not propelling ourselves through the sea as fish do by weaving—we are nonetheless, like fish, moving without the use of limbs. In so doing, we enter the vastness of geologic time.

By calling attention to our bones, weight-resistance yoga practice, in general, and spinal exercises, in particular, evoke not only our past as primitive vertebrates but our future as mere skeletons. Perhaps 380 millions years hence, in some new geological age, our fossils may be found in sedimentary rock, an asphalt deposit, coal, or amber—an exciting discovery of the past made by a future generation in the dark about its own past. (Fossils weren't generally recognized as remains of living things from our distant past until about 1800.) More likely, though, our bones will turn to dust.

The weight-resistance yogin's consideration of the skeleton is a contemplation on the propinquity of death. A contemplation that centers not on the abstract truth of death, nor even on an image of death, nor even (morbidly and sentimentally) on a foul, decaying corpse left out (i.e., not buried) in charnel grounds, but on the cool, tangible presence of our death within us: our bones. The entire weight-resistance yoga practice, in its rejection of the most elementary human inclinations, may be said to be a contemplation of death. But this is especially so of the trunk exercises.

In our everyday lives, we're infatuated—and rightly so!—by what we find alluring. But in the weight-resistance yoga session, we perceive that what arouses strong desire in us—and much else—isn't lasting. We experience the poignancy of our mortality. We know in our very bones what scholar-practitioner of tantra yoga Stuart Sovatsky describes as "our finite segment of the eternal." This comprehension directs us toward fully inhabiting the fleeting present.[1]

On Nonviolence

Back Raise

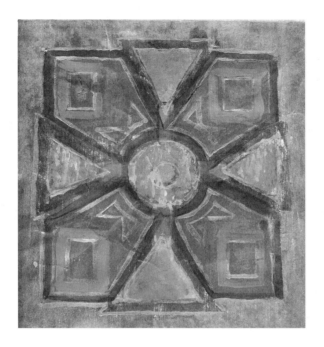

One side [which is overstretched] thus manifests deliberate violence,
and the other side [which is understretched], non-deliberate violence.

—B. K. S. IYENGAR, *THE TREE OF YOGA*

The upward phase of the back raise, the strengthening exercise performed while lying face down on the Roman chair, resembles Bhujangasana, Cobra Pose. In this position, I think of myself not as a cobra in a dense highland forest but as a seahorse bobbing around in sea grass meadows, mangrove stands, or coral reefs. However they're imagined, though, these exercises that extend the back are commonly feared (and condemned) for putting the lower back in danger: applying high compressive forces to the lumbar spine risks damage to its joints, ligaments and discs. Back extension is controlled primarily by the erector spinae muscles, the three columns of muscles (the iliocostalis, longissimus dorsi, and spinalis dorsi) that originate on the sacrum and lower spine and insert on the ribs, upper spine, and skull.

165

While stretching anterior muscles (the rectus femoris, rectus abdominis, obliques, pectoralis major, and others) by lengthening them, Bhujangasana also strengthens posterior spinal muscles by shortening them. The Roman-chair back raise, which targets the lower-back muscles for strengthening, is considered more dangerous than this pose. Although it opens up the front of the body nearly to the same extent as Bhujangasana, it applies considerably more compressive force to the lumbar spine because the lower back is more isolated and exposed to the pull of gravity.

The real danger to the lumbar spine during the Roman-chair back raise, however, lies not in the exercise per se but in performing the exercise with poor form. Some weight lifters fully relax in the bent-over position (when the extensor muscles are allowed to go limp, they become electronically silent, or totally at rest); lurch up (when the back is snapped up, the extensor muscles are shocked into action); and lift the pelvis (when the axis of rotation moves to the hips, the back hyperextends). These weight lifters also tend to overtrain (perform too many sets) and fail to adapt progressively (they hold a heavy weight to their chest from the get-go instead of gradually increasing the weight load over a period of time). Performing the Roman chair exercise in any of these ways risks injury. It's what B. K. S. Iyengar describes as active, or deliberate, violence.

Nervous about applying an unaccustomed workload to their back by moving through a wide range of motion against gravity, other weight lifters (even those who are fit adults) do the Roman-chair exercise timidly. They use a greatly constricted range of motion, keeping their back splinted, barely moving down or up. The erector spinae in the lumbar region is most efficiently strengthened by moving the back in a succession of curlings and uncurlings by rounding the back (in the downward phase) and arching the lower back (in the upward phase). (At the lumbar spine, this folding and unfolding is a reverse of the abdominal curl.)

And if these weight lifters hold a weight to add to the resistance, it's usually a light one. While everyday lifting activities call for this caution, strength training doesn't. For a muscle to increase in strength, the stress to which it's subjected during an exercise must be increased beyond what it normally undergoes. Muscles adapt to unaccustomed stress—an increase in work load—by becoming progressively stronger (this phenomenon is called the overload principle).

A strong erector spinae muscle group is needed in everyday life to keep the vertebral spine aligned, arch the back, and support the trunk, not to mention carry out back-lifting activities. Trunk extension in lifting is usually a compound movement, carried out by both lumbar and hip (gluteal and hamstring) extensors. But because the more powerful hip muscles are responsible for most of the movement, over time a muscle imbalance is created that leaves the lumbar muscles weak. Rarely isolated during everyday activities, lumbar extensors need to encounter the overload provided by a weight-resistance exercise allocated solely to them in order to gain the strength required to prevent low-back injury.

Performing the back raise timorously thwarts any increase in the capacity of the lumbar extensors to generate greater force. An undemanding practice promotes deconditioning, which leads to deterioration of the joint structures. Iyengar describes performing an exercise in these ways as passive, or nondeliberate, violence: "Though it may appear non-violent, it is also violence as the cells will die when they do not perform their functions as they should."[2]

So, as we see, fretting about the safety of weight-resistance (and weight-surrender) exercises may sometimes be self-destructive: the neurotic need to perform strengthening exercises cautiously would produce maladaptation, while risky training would lead to successful adaptation. Only a Roman-chair-back-extension exercise that rolls the back down to nearly full flexion (without relaxation) and carefully unrolls the back one vertebra at a time to full extension (without engaging the hips) at a sufficiently high intensity is useful for lower back pain prevention, rehabilitation, and maintenance. As contrarian fitness guru Mel C. Siff argues: "[T]he body will adapt to certain levels of 'harmful' exercising, provided that this is not imposed near the mechanical limits of the given soft tissues. If this is done progressively in a controlled manner, then the body should become capable of handling all of the so-called dangerous activity."[3] Performing an exercise in this way is neither overdoing nor underdoing it. The exercise is carried out with nonviolence—what in yoga is called *ahimsa*.

When we achieve ahimsa in weight-resistance yoga, we gain more than nonviolence against the body. Embodied in our actions, nonviolence is transferred to our everyday lives—especially to our relationships with our loved ones. We neither get bitterly angry with them nor passively give in to them. We don't wish them harm or wish they'd go away, or feel offended, wronged, or mis-treated by them. We keep in mind our love for them. In the presence of our non-violence, hostility and resentment are avoided—whether belonging to us or to others.

And if it's too late—if, whether reacting to or causing anger in others, we've already seized hold of anger and wielded it like a heavy stick—by firmly re-grounding ourselves in nonviolence, we create the conditions for us and others to let go of the anger. We make reconciliation possible. This is what Patanjali meant, I think, when he observed in the *Yoga Sutras* (translated by the yogin and scholar Ernest E. Wood with his usual practicality and psychological insight): "When non-injury is accomplished, there will be abandonment of animosity in [our] presence."[4]

On Withdrawal
Ab Curl

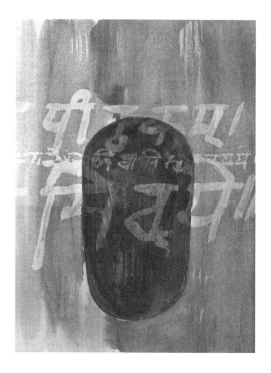

Indifference to worldly enjoyments is very difficult to obtain.
—Svatmarama, *The Hatha Yoga Pradipika*

Our routine breathing is not only shallow but also uneven, a reflection of a mind that's disordered, even if only slightly so. Traditional yogic meditation seeks to deepen and regulate breathing as a means to order the mind. Yet, while yogic deep breathing calms the mind, it stirs the body. During yogic meditative practice, as the mind turns quiet, the body sings.

During intense strengthening exercises, in contrast, almost right from the start the body is energized by exertion, and breathing is forced. As the demand increases for oxygen consumption and carbon dioxide removal in the working muscles, the breathing of most weight lifters goes out of control: haphazard, spasmodic, and labored, the breath turns into gasping and heaving. Weight-resistance yogins rein in this wild breath.

When desperate for air, we have difficulty enough breathing evenly and continuously; but weight-resistance yogins breathe through the nose, making the task yet more difficult. (Breathing through the nose requires three times as much energy as breathing through the nose and mouth—that is, it's three times more difficult.) With determination and concentration, however, slow, rhythmic, deep nasal breathing can be maintained. Accomplished practitioners use the *ujjayi* breath. It's performed by breathing in and out through both nostrils while constricting the throat (more specifically, partially closing the glottis), resulting in a sound that some liken to a deep hissing but I think of as the roll of ocean waves on the shore. Beginners are better off using the *sitkari* breath, which involves inhaling through a slightly opened mouth with a relaxed tongue and exhaling through the nose.

Quiet breathing, when the body is at rest, is performed by the primary inspiratory muscles—the intercostals, scalenes, and diaphragm. The contraction of the intercostals and scalenes pull on the rib cage to expand the thorax, allowing the lungs contained within it to expand and draw in fresh atmospheric air. Meanwhile, the diaphragm, a dome-shaped muscle that divides the thorax and abdomen, contracts downward, flattening out. Expiration is passive. The intercostals, scalenes and diaphragm just relax, allowing the thorax—and thus the lungs—to return to resting size. Foul air passes out into the atmosphere.

During deep, or forced, breathing, previously dormant muscles are recruited to meet the increased demands of expiration. The abdominal muscles (transversus abdominis, internal oblique abdominal, external oblique abdominal, and rectus abdominis) play a critical role in forced expiration. When they contract, they pull the ribs toward the back. The resultant rise in pressure inside the abdominal cavity pushes the diaphragm up into the thoracic cage. The vertical space of the thorax decreased, air is forcefully expelled from the lungs.

When we consider the abdominals in light of this critical contribution to the process of deep breathing (as well as their other functions: stabilizing, flexing, and rotating the trunk; compressing the abdominal contents during coughing, sneezing, vomiting, and straining to lift; bearing down during urination, defecation, and parturition; and pulling on the front of the pelvis to prevent lower back strain), we realize what ninnies we are to get caught up in wanting to sculpt a soft tummy into a tight, well-defined anterior abdominal wall for display.

When we stop desiring (or ogling) cut washboard "abs"—which means to say, when we become less concerned about our appearance—we take a step on our spiritual path. As yoga scholar Mircea Eliade comments, "We should note that it is by stages that the yogin dissociates himself from life. He begins by suppressing the least essential habits of living—comforts, distractions, waste of time, dispersion of his mental forces, etc. He then attempts to unify the most important functions of life—respiration, consciousness."[5] Unifying respiration and consciousness leads us to recognize the unity of all things.

Although it appears that when we inhale we're actively taking in air (especially when, under exertion, we're gasping for breath), in actuality, we're not pulling in air at all. Air flows toward areas of lower pressure. When the diaphragm contracts, the volume of the thoracic cavity increases, causing the air pressure in the lungs to fall below the atmospheric pressure. Air simply flows from the region of high pressure (the atmosphere) into the region of low pressure (our chest cavity). In this manner, air is drawn into (and subsequently forced out of) the lungs.

We ordinarily think of ourselves as a solitary self (constructed over the course of our life) distinct from the world. But awareness of our breath reminds us of our interdependence with the atmosphere that surrounds us and envelops all of Earth. And, by extension, it reminds us of our connection to Earth, whose gravitational field retains the gaseous mass that makes up the atmosphere, and to all the celestial bodies beyond Earth's atmosphere, swirling in the heavens. In mindful breathing, the usual distinctions between observer and observed, subject and object, self and world dissolve. Weight-resistance yoga practice becomes a withdrawal from profane life and an entrance into a life that places the body not only in rhythm with the breath but with the cosmos. Om!

18

MEDITATIONS ON THE HIP JOINT AND PELVIC GIRDLE

■ On Stability—Introduction to the Hip Joint and Pelvic Girdle

The standing human body is stable when its line of gravity falls within its base of support: namely, our two feet and the area between them. Stability becomes increasingly precarious as our center of gravity nears the edge of our base. When the line of gravity falls outside our feet, we fall.

■ On Standing Up—Bent-Leg Hip Extension and Hanging Knee Raise

If we think about the mechanics of rising at all, it's probably because our ability to stand (or the ability of someone close to us) has been impaired or even lost. During the weight-resistance yoga session, when we reflect on what it means to be human, we consider how standing up is a critical aspect not only of our daily life and the evolutionary development of our species but also the biological development of the individual.

■ On Arrested Falling—Hip Abduction and Hip Adduction

While not an act of derring-do, like that of a tightrope walker crossing a high wire, the simple act of walking on the ground is, when you think about it, an amazing balancing act all the same. A rhythmical movement in which the center of gravity is swung forward, human bipedal gait places us in peril at every step.

On Stability

Introduction to the Hip Joint and Pelvic Girdle

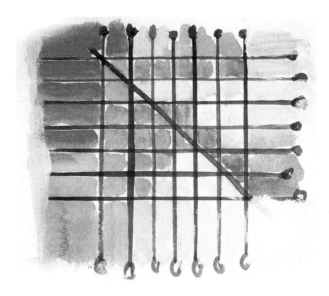

By cultivating gladness for those who are happy, compassion for those who are suffering, delight in those who are kind-hearted and disregard toward those who are selfish and mean, we habitually remain calm.

—Patanjali: *Yoga Sutras*

An object's center of gravity—the place where Earth's gravity is considered to act on the object—is the point at which its mass is concentrated. Located within the object (say, a hard-boiled egg, a baseball bat, or an automobile), but not usually coinciding with its geometric center, the center of gravity can be approximated by finding the object's balance point, the place where the object can be twirled about (at least theoretically) on one finger.

In the anatomic position (standing upright with the palms of the hands forward), the human body's center of gravity—the point around which the body's mass is evenly distributed—lies approximately just in front of the second sacral vertebra. (The precise location depends on our height, weight, and frame—our unique proportions.)

If our body is fixed in this position, then no matter how it's angled to

Earth—whether standing upright, leaning, lying, or standing upside down—our center of gravity doesn't change. (Picture the prone, unbending silent movie comic Buster Keaton, quiet and dignified, seemingly gliding through the air as he grasps onto the back of a moving cable car.) What produces a new center of gravity is movement of a body segment (say, lifting a leg to give a ball a hard kick).

The line of gravity—the action line of the force of gravity on an object—is like a plumb line attached to the center of gravity. Regardless of the orientation of the object on Earth (including in its atmosphere), the line of gravity is always vertically downward toward the center of Earth. For an object to be stable, the line of gravity must fall within the object's base of support.

The standing human body is stable when its line of gravity falls within its base of support: namely our two feet and the area between them. Stability becomes increasingly precarious as our center of gravity nears the edge of our base. When the line of gravity falls outside our feet, we fall.

In everyday life, of course, we seldom stand rigidly for long. We move. And we're moved. Gravity is the most consistent external force encountered by the human body, but there are others: objects that we're wearing, carrying, or using pull on us; strong winds, ocean waves, and other natural elements buffet us about; and people push or pull us. We can increase our stability (give our line of gravity more freedom to move without falling outside its base of support) in response to these external forces by lowering our center of gravity (by bending our knees) and/or by making our base of support larger (by widening our stance or by relying on the support of a cane, a walker, crutches, a ballet barre, or the like), heavier (by adding ballast to our legs), and stronger (by performing strengthening exercises for the lower body, including our hips).

The hip joint consists of the ball-like head of the upper leg bone (the femur) and the hip socket (acetabulum) of the pelvic girdle. The pelvic girdle consists of the right and left pelvic bones joined together posteriorly by the sacrum (the triangular bone at the base of the spine) and anteriorly by the pubic bones. Although favoring stability over mobility, the hip joint is the second most mobile joint (after the shoulder joint) in the body. Routine movement of the hip joint usually involves movement of the pelvic girdle. For example, in walking, hip flexion (lifting the leg forward) is accompanied by pelvic girdle forward rotation (anterior tilt), and hip extension (bringing the leg backward) is accompanied by pelvic girdle backward rotation (posterior tilt).

Weight-resistance yogins faithfully strengthen the four major groups of hip muscles: the flexors (which move the upper leg straight forward and up), the extensors (which move the upper leg straight backward and up), the abductors (which move the upper leg to the side away from the midline), and the adductors (which move the upper leg from the side toward the midline). Most of these muscles also act as external rotators (which rotate the upper leg away from the midline) or internal rotators (which rotate the upper leg toward the midline).

As we age, we come to consider the importance of having strong and healthy hips. As we've seen, the hips (along with the other segments of the lower body) counteract the pull of gravity and the effect of other forces and allow us to be ambulatory, as well as act as a pillar that supports the trunk and head. But we who practice weight-resistance yoga also recognize how an embodied practice that includes exercises that strengthen the hips, perhaps especially in their role as stabilizers, can help change our behavior—which means to say, shape the self.

Many of us are ruled by uncontrollable patterns of behavior that make us unhappy. Yet they seem to us to be rational responses to people around us and events out of our control. Put upon, we become irritable and fly off the handle. Feeling slighted, we sulk, nursing the desire to get even. Feeling unappreciated, we constantly seek acknowledgment. When expectations go awry, we lose heart or turn cynical and pessimistic. Our center is unstable.

Through working on hip-strengthening exercises, weight-resistance yogins attain a physical stability that overtime comes to correspond to an inner stability—a stability that isn't a steady condition impervious to the world but an engaged response to the world. We embrace others. We seek their embrace. Yet we detach ourselves from their crazy talk. We retain our equanimity. When we're "pushed" and "pulled" by sudden, unforeseen events, large and small, we're not upended. We receive good news and bad news, success and failure equably. We remain calm and undisturbed. Sometimes we teeter. But grounded in the earth (through accommodation with gravity) and yearning for the heavens (through resisting gravity and standing upright), we soon move back to our vital center.

On Standing Up

Bent-Leg Hip Extension and Hanging Knee Raise

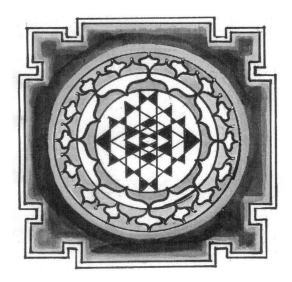

To know is accordingly the ability to stand in the manifestness of things that exist, to endure them. Merely to have information, however abundant, is not to know.

—MARTIN HEIDEGGER, *AN INTRODUCTION TO METAPHYSICS*

Bring a leg back. This movement—hip extension—is performed by the large gluteal muscles, which make up the buttocks. Feel your buttocks. Although layered over with fat, the gluteus maximus, which forms most of the muscle of the buttocks, is easily palpable. That's because it originates on the posterior spine and pelvis and inserts on the upper leg. Bring the leg forward and up. This movement—hip flexion—is primarily performed by the iliopsoas, which lifts the leg beyond the normal standing position. Moving obliquely from the small of the back through the pelvic bowl to attach at the front upper leg, the iliopsoas, although large, is palpable only in the emaciated or in the thin who relax their abdominal muscles and have evacuated their bowels.

These two dissimilar and opposing muscles—the gluteus maximus and iliopsoas—work together sequentially, sometimes in an alternating rhythm, to perform a variety of motions that require strong anterior/posterior action of the hips.

They contract during jumping and leaping. They provide action to propel the body forward when walking up an incline, such as a ramp or hill. When climbing stairs, while the gluteal muscles work to shift the body's weight over the supporting leg, the iliopsoas works to lift the swinging leg. Both muscles play a critical role in running, not only in propelling the body forward but also in stabilizing the body to keep it from pitching over. Although they aren't strongly contracted during ordinary walking, the gluteal muscles and iliopsoas are strongly brought into play in another common daily activity: standing up from sitting.

In general, we prefer sitting to standing. The act of sitting down, especially as we get older, is a pleasurable activity. It sometimes produces a sigh of relief. We're equipped for sitting. Compared to ape buttocks, human buttocks are quite large. Apes sit on their ischial tuberosities, sitz bones, which protrude through their fur; we're cushioned by prominent rounded buttocks. Aristotle observed:

> The posterior bottom of the trunk and the parts about the upper legs are peculiar in man as compared with quadrupeds. Nearly all these latter have a tail. But man is tailless. He has, however, fleshy buttocks, which don't exist in quadrupeds. His thighs are also fleshy. There is one explanation: of all animals, man alone stands erect. Standing causes no fatigue to quadrupeds, and even the long continuance of this posture produces in them no weariness; for they are supported the whole time by four props, which is much as though they were lying down. But for man, it's no easy task to remain for any length of time on his feet; his body demands rest in a sitting position. This, then, is the reason why man has fleshy buttocks and thighs.[1]

But, sooner or later, stand up we must. In fact, rising to a standing position from a sitting position is one of the most critical activities of daily life. Just consider early morning before we go out in the world: we get out of bed, get up from the toilet seat, and leave our chair at the kitchen table after breakfast.

Rising from a seat involves four phases. In the first phase, to initiate momentum for rising, we lean forward as we fix our upper legs, shifting the center of gravity of the trunk over our feet. In the second phase, in order to transfer momentum to the whole body, as we leave the seat we slightly bend our knees. In the third phase, we begin to straighten the knees, hips, and trunk as the body rises. In the fourth phase, we stabilize the body in the full upright position. The first and second phases recruit the iliopsoas; the third phase, the gluteal muscles; and the fourth stage, both.

If we think about the mechanics of rising at all, it's probably because our ability to stand (or the ability of someone close to us) has been impaired or even lost. During the weight-resistance yoga session, when we reflect on what it means to be human, we consider how standing up is a critical aspect not only of our daily life and the evolutionary development of our species but also the biological development of the individual. In first standing up without support, the child has no concern for security. Failure—falling down—doesn't discourage the child one bit. The forceful urge to get up, to resist downward-pulling forces—while in a state of precarious balance!—overcomes any fear. "In getting up," observes German phenomenological psychologist Irwin W. Straus, a child "gains his standing in the world. The parents are not the only ones who greet the child's progress with joy. The child enjoys no less the triumph of his achievement."[2] There's no need for parental attention, yet applause.

Fitness trainers regularly use the parenting model of "providing positive feedback" with their clients. This training philosophy of "bolstering self-esteem" fosters an inappropriate relationship: some semblance of parent/child and even lover/beloved or sadist/masochist. (A relationship largely formed, it might be said, in order to reinforce a chimerical and superficial goal: looking good.)

In contrast, yoga teachers, including weight-resistance yoga teachers, don't shore up self-esteem and provide positive reinforcement. They don't get caught up in praise (and its implicit threat: the withdrawal of praise—which means to say, blame. They don't provide motivation by cajoling, scolding, or goading students. They don't chitchat; there's too much to attend to. They simply demonstrate correct form to students and then correct students' form by making adjustments, thereby aiding students in moving deeper into an exercise.

Of course, weight-resistance yoga teachers do much else. They set a tone—from mindful to devotional—for the session. They help us recognize how our movements reveal our habitual thoughts, emotions, and attitudes, so we can discard those that interfere with our spiritual path. They aid us in becoming fully absorbed in our movements as a means of accessing realities beyond everyday life. But no matter how much they guide us, we always know that it's through our own self-discipline that our life is transformed and that it's only we—in part through our reverent and upright posture—who can open ourselves up to the ground of Being.

On Arrested Falling
Hip Abduction and Hip Adduction

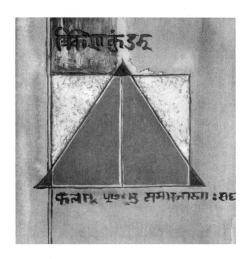

In yoga we do well to avoid too much of the idea that we are bound to the earth, even physically . . . [T]he earth pulls us towards it by gravity, but we also pull it upwards to us, also by gravity. We thus have a share of the original power, and when walking . . . we do to some extent float.

—ERNEST WOOD, *YOGA DICTIONARY*

Between five and six million years ago, a new type of primate evolved in Eastern Africa—one that walked on two legs instead of ambling along on all fours with its front knuckles to the ground. Bipedalism was literally the first evolutionary step that divided hominids from apes. To develop the ability to walk upright, the anatomy of our ancestors underwent complex changes that shifted the upper body over the pelvis and the lower body more directly under the pelvis. (Recent research has shown that some aspects of human anatomy may have evolved in order to accommodate running, not walking.)

Among the changes that took place was the angling inward toward the body's midline of the thighbone (femur) as it slopes toward the knee. In apes, the femur runs straight down from hip to knee, which accounts for their boxy, side-to-side, swaying gait. Humans are wider in the hips than through the knees, which improves our balance. As is our wont, we've used this mechanical advantage to individualize our gait.

As you walk down a sidewalk in a shopping area in springtime, note how the sway of people's hips varies, depending on their frame, age, speed, and mood, as well as their status and personality. As Mabel E. Todd, one of the pioneers of bodywork, observed in 1937: "Watch any man as he walks down the avenue, and you can determine his status in life. With practice, a finer discernment will have him placed socially and economically, and with a fair idea of his outlook on life."[3]

Even those of us with little discernment of body language have noticed (if only in some vague way) that a person's gait is expressive of his or her emotional make-up. A genial disposition, a touchy temperament, strong or weak character, a pinched or expansive personality, meek or overbearing behavior are all, we'd agree, expressed in gait. But whatever a person's unique gait, the mechanics of his or her walking are the same. Walking consists of a swing phase and a support phase.

Slip behind a woman wearing tight jeans and take a dispassionate look, if possible, at the changes in the position of her hips made with each step. (Because women's hips are generally wider then men's, a woman's gait is more pronounced, making it a more advantageous subject of study.) Note that when her right leg lifts off the ground, during the beginning of the swing phase, she's standing on her left leg. The right side of her pelvis is unsupported, leaving her vulnerable to tipping over to the right. What keeps her from falling over?

During the swing phase, the abductors (the group of hip muscles that attach to the upper, outside part of the leg) of the supporting (left) leg contract to oppose the tendency of the pelvis to drop on the unsupported (right) side. At the same time, the adductors (the group of hip muscles that attach to the leg on the inside of the thigh) of the swinging (right) leg contract to shift the pelvis over, moving the upper body weight over the supporting (left) leg. The right leg lifts (bends at the knee) and then straightens (extends at the knee). The swing phase ends as the heel of the right foot is placed on the ground. When the whole foot is placed flat on the ground, the hip adductors and abductors of both legs stabilize the pelvis. This support phase ends when the heel of the trailing (left) leg is raised in push off.

While not an act of derring-do, like that of a tightrope walker crossing a high wire, this simple act of walking on the ground is, when you think about it, an amazing balancing act all the same. A rhythmical movement in which the center of gravity is swung forward, human bipedal gait places us in peril at every step. As we've seen, the whole weight of the body rests for a short time on only one leg, destabilizing the body, thereby putting us at risk of falling—until the leg brought forward reaches the ground, once again rescuing us from the threatened fall. As phenomenological psychologist Erwin W. Straus observed: "Human gait is, in fact, a continuously arrested falling."[4]

For this reason, it can be said that walking is an assumptive act: upon taking a step, we take for granted that the leg brought forward will ultimately find solid ground, and that we won't fall. We might trip over an unseen obstacle or unevenness of ground. Somebody might knock us over. Our weak or frail bones might precipitate a collapse. But, by and large, we're not anxious when we walk. Most of the time, our experience of walking is pedestrian: we move from Point A to Point B without any worries.

Which is all the more reason to keep the hip joints strong and healthy. A marvel of locomotive engineering, the hips lose their effectiveness as we age. By strengthening the hip muscles—in particular, the two hip abductors, the gluteus medius and gluteus minimus—twice a week during weight-resistance yoga sessions, we can, to a great degree, retain the spring of youth in our step. This strengthening will allow us to continue putting one leg in front of the other to ambulate without giving a thought to it. Not that attentiveness to walking is a bad thing.

Hatha yoga praises the body—not so that we can display it as a proud possession, but so that we can use it to remain still during seated meditation (when we forget the body) or to move with steadiness and ease during the moving meditations of weight-surrender and weight-resistance yoga (when we remember the body). Without a fit and healthy body, we cannot know bliss. But the physical conditioning aspect of hatha yoga doesn't benefit only these periods set aside from everyday life for achieving altered states; it also makes possible transportive experiences during everyday life, such as walking down the street, perhaps on one of those days when it's lightly raining and the fragrance of trees is strong.

As we effortlessly stroll along, we turn our attention to our stride: the swing phase and the stability phase feel so secure and coordinated and elegant, they seem to be acting through us. By this I mean that we can't identify the doer. We don't make decisions about taking steps. They just happen. "We" are no more doing the walking than "it" is raining. There's no will to move or submission to being moved. There's just serenely happy walking.

19

MEDITATIONS
ON THE KNEE JOINT

▪ On Pain—Introduction to the Knee Joint

Performed correctly (at a rather high intensity), weight-resistance yoga exercises are painful. But weight-resistance yogins are attentive to all aspects of exercises, even to the pain—perhaps, especially to the pain. We constantly monitor any discomfort, distinguishing between a brittle pain, an indication that the exercise should be stopped to prevent injury, and a sturdy pain, an indication of muscle strengthening.

▪ On Calmness—Prone Knee Curl and Knee Extension

I believe that there is a training benefit to maintaining a calm expression. Contorting the face detracts from correctly performing quadriceps and hamstring (and other) exercises because it disperses concentration. Having a calm face is a spur for fully focusing on the contraction of the targeted muscles.

On Pain

Introduction to the Knee Joint

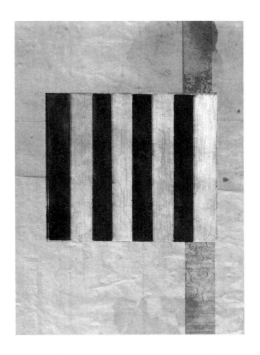

As the forward stretching is sustained, the complaining mind learns to surrender to the discomfort felt in the legs and in the back. This surrender can become a doorway to a quiet world within the body.

—Jean Couch with Nell Weaver,
Runner's World Yoga Book

Performed correctly (at a rather high intensity), weight-resistance yoga exercises are painful. Particularly painful are two machine exercises for the knees: the knee extension and the prone knee curl. The knee extension exercise involves elevating the lower legs against resistance while seated, which primarily strengthens the quadriceps femoris. The prone knee curl exercise involves bringing the lower legs up against resistance while lying face down, which primarily strengthens the hamstrings.

We can lessen the pain of these exercises by several mechanical means: using a lighter resistance; limiting the range of motion; flinging up the resistance with momentum; and lurching (by recruiting lower back muscles) to initiate the motion. However, because they lessen the optimal tension for the muscles most involved, all of these means make the exercises inefficient—and the last two risk injury.

We can also lessen the pain of these exercises by distracting ourselves—listening to music, talking to a trainer, or simply letting our mind wander. But weight-resistance yogins are attentive to all aspects of exercises, even to the pain—perhaps, especially to the pain. If only for safety's sake, we constantly monitor any discomfort, distinguishing between a brittle pain (one that is often sharp, thin, and tinny), an indication that the exercise should be stopped to prevent injury, and a sturdy pain (one that incrementally becomes full and resonant and is commonly likened to a burning sensation), an indication of muscle strengthening.

There's no getting around it. The presence of pain is an inescapable part of weight-resistance yoga training.

For over 300 years, the dominant explanation of pain derived from René Descartes, who posited in 1664 that an injury stimulates specific nerves, which transport an impulse to the brain, producing pain "just as, pulling on one end of a cord, one simultaneously rings a bell which hangs at the opposite end."[1] But this mechanical explanation doesn't take into account that people experience pain differently: some have a higher threshold and tolerance for pain than others.

Driven, self-disciplined, and fit, ballet dancers are inured to pain. They perform through sprains and stress fractures (and, as a result, commonly develop long-term injuries). Soldiers report slight or no pain from injuries that routinely require narcotics in civilians. Clearly, dancers and soldiers diminish or even banish the sensation of pain by recontextualizing it.

Weight-resistance yogins also cope with pain by recontextualizing it. We know that pain is ordinarily the result of an injury or disease; whether great and constant or slight and intermittent, this unelected pain is without value (some things in life do happen in vain and to think otherwise is a kind of magical thinking). The pain of weight-resistance yoga, in contrast, isn't without point: it's endured in the service of achieving strength fitness. Accordingly, we modify our response to the pain. We know that complaining about it would be as foolish (and unseemly) as grumbling—"whining" is more like it—about having to compromise with our husband or wife or having to sacrifice for our children. Yet sometimes we still find ourselves bitterly complaining.

When this happens, we do something else to cope with pain: we closely observe the coming and going of our aversion responses to it—all that complaining we're so quick to do. *I hate this. I resent this. I wish this were over. I wish this would go away.* In separating our aversion responses from the pain sensations themselves, we realize (once we've committed ourselves to doing the exercises) that pain may come and go. It's out of our control. But our psychomental responses to pain, in contrast, can be controlled. We're not compelled to act on them or even entertain them. We can take them or leave them. In this way, we come to relinquish the desire to flee from or even alleviate pain.

Consequently, we go about our routine without complaint—not out of compliance or stoicism, but because there's nothing to complain about. I think this is what Couch and Weaver mean when they assert that surrendering to discomfort by giving up noisily complaining about it (even silently to ourselves!) allows us to find a "quiet world within the body."[2]

With its emphasis on observing our habitual attitude toward pain during the exercise session, weight-resistance yoga provides us with an opportunity for altering our response not only to pain but also to suffering. In recognizing that the sensation of pain is distinct from our aversion response to it, we come to see that it's this aversion response that constitutes suffering. Our suffering ends when we realize that our aversion responses (like our pleasure responses) are separate from our true self.

Through undergoing this process in the exercise session, weight-resistance yogins model a behavior that helps us accept life's hardships—economic misfortune, political oppression, missed opportunities, loss of loved ones, disease, and old age—without suffering. We know that suffering serves no purpose and is simply bare suffering, without meaning. The German psychotherapist and Zen master Karlfried Graf Von Dürckheim observes: "The calm bearing of the meditating monk reminds men that to suffer from life shows only estrangement from life."[3]

On Calmness
Prone Knee Curl and Knee Extension

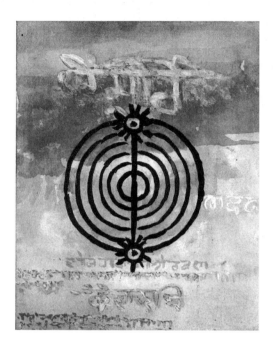

When I wasn't catching any fish, my father used to tell me I wasn't holding my mouth right.

—John Jerome, *The Sweet Spot in Time*

In performing our exercises, weight-resistance yogins place particular emphasis on bringing the body into a stillness out of which all movement is generated. During both the knee extension exercise, which targets the quadriceps muscles, and the knee curl exercise, which targets the hamstring muscles, the trunk and hips are stabilized. While seated during the knee extension, we don't rock to fling our legs up. While lying belly down during the leg curl, we don't twitch to thrust our legs back. These extraneous movements—cheating motions—help move the resistance but undermine our strengthening goals. The targeted muscles are underutilized.

In addition to fixating a joint so that the desired movement can be performed at another joint, we also relax those parts of the body with no influence on the contraction of the muscles most involved in the joint movement. "You can release greater energy to the isolated muscle by learning to relax your other body parts," maintains Ellington Darden, a disciple of Arthur Jones, the inventor of Nautilus exercise equipment. "This allows for more efficient growth stimulation."[4] Scrunching up our shoulders, rolling on our heels, or excessively gripping the handles wastes energy. "Even tensing the jaws [and] squinting the eyes," Darden argues, "can weaken the neurological input to a given area of the body."[5] More than any other exercises, knee extensions and knee curls cry out for contorting the face from strain.

There are tips for preventing tension from forming in the face during a strenuous exercise. First, relax tense surrounding muscles located in the shoulder and neck (including the throat). Then, close the mouth. Unclench the teeth. Allow tightened jaw to drop without opening the mouth. Relax the tongue so that it lies limply on the mouth floor. Relax the lips, the flesh surrounding the mouth and nostrils, the cheeks, the frowning brows—the entire face.

When all is said and done, though, is relaxing the face really necessary to preserve energy? I'm skeptical. Almost surely, the waste of energy of the grimace on the contraction of the quadriceps or hamstring muscles is minimal or nonexistent. I believe, however, that there is a training benefit to maintaining a calm expression. Contorting the face detracts from correctly performing quadriceps and hamstring (and other) exercises because it disperses concentration. Having a calm face is a spur for fully focusing on the contraction of the targeted muscles. Not that there aren't other reasons, ones less directly related to making strength gains, for maintaining a placid expression.

In his 1940 strength-training manual *Physique & Figure*, the famed Indian bodybuilder K. V. Iyer counseled:

> Do not strain or contract your face, however difficult the movement may be, or however strongly you may be flexing the muscles. There must not be even a twitch of the muscle on the face, no gritting of the teeth, no biting of the nether lip, no knotting of the brows. In short, while the flexion of the particular muscle or group of muscles should be very, very intense, the face should be normal and calm while exercising. It is even better if the face assumes a soft smile instead of being cold or hard.[6]

Iyer gave this advice to his students to help them develop grace. He valued "the graceful movement of the limbs while exercising" over all other aspects of strength training. "Not that you should swing and sway to music," he cautioned, "but while you are using your limbs for exercises let them be used as gracefully as possible." He considered maintaining a calm expression as a critical aspect of being graceful. "There should be nothing ugly or contortioned either in your movements or in the facial expression. You should develop this quality [grace] to the fullest extent possible."[7]

Important as obtaining grace is, however, I believe that there's another, altogether different and more important, reason for maintaining a calm expression during strength-training exercises: it facilitates withdrawing from the everyday world and turning inward.

Most of us wouldn't want a face that's restless or rigid. We prefer a face that's in complete repose. Yet we also want that face to be instantly capable of expressing nuances of feeling and even volatile emotions—excitability, anxiety, rage, grief. A face, in other words, that reflects the subtlety and depth of our emotions.

But in the weight-resistance yoga session, we observe tapas, or asceticism—which extends to our facial expressiveness. Whereas ordinarily we eagerly display our feelings to others, in the weight-resistance yoga session, just as we're absent words and gestures that reveal our thoughts and feelings, we're absent facial expressions that reveal our thoughts and feelings. We make our face into a mask. As the Indian philosopher Vācaspati Miśra understood, this mask is a sign of great self-mastery: "The absence of facial indications, by which the inner secrets of the mind are revealed, constitutes control over oneself, so that thought is not communicated by chance and to anyone at random."[8] In assuming opaqueness during the weight-resistance yoga session, we act in solitude.

Not that our intention is to be antisocial. It's just that our entire life isn't normal during hatha yoga practice. During this time, we grandly oppose the most elemental human inclinations: not only the need to connect to others but also the impulse to move unthinkingly, breathe unevenly, and stir up our emotions, which may be reflected in our face. Instead, we make deliberate movements within a static position, breathe rhythmically, and fully concentrate—thus emptying and calming the mind, which is reflected in a relaxed and blank face. Then, we find that we are no longer hiding our disordered emotions. We simply don't have them. In this way, our complex and fragmented everyday life is replaced by a mode of being that's simplified and unified. We're whole. And as a result, serenity is bestowed upon us.

MEDITATIONS ON THE ANKLE JOINT

■ **On Motion—Introduction to the Ankle Joint**

The six simple machines are the lever, pulley, wheel and axle, inclined plane, wedge, and screw. Of these, the lever alone was made in humankind's image. For it may be said that the human body is a system of levers. We who invented the lever are ourselves a hodgepodge of seesaws, crowbars, balance scales, nutcrackers, wheelbarrows, screen doors (operated by a short spring), catapults, and other levers.

■ **On Pleasurable Repetition—Standing Heel Raise,**
  Seated Heel Raise, and Weighted Toe Raise

During weight-resistance yoga practice, you might say that the body itself is retelling or reenacting the same story by repeating the same movements: the story of making old things new. Just as when our eyes become accustomed to the darkness in a room, we see the room fill up with objects, when we set ourselves to doing a weight-resistance exercise exactly so, we find that we notice all the rich details demanded by the exercise. And then, most astonishingly: the exercise becomes new, as if we were doing it for the first time.

On Motion

Introduction to the Ankle Joint

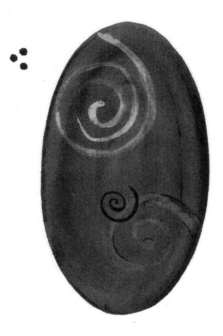

[Prof. Iyer] would open up and disassemble any appliance he brought home in order to understand the innards, and then reassemble it. He had great interest in repairing electrical appliances, especially radios and tape recorders. It is not surprising that he who wanted to understand the secrets of the body also wanted to discern the secrets of appliances, too.

—A. R. MITHRA, ED., *PROF. K. V. IYER: A REMEMBRANCE*

Our notion of a machine is usually some wondrous early-industrial-age contraption—a diesel engine, say, or a steam turbine—some machine with complex, interrelated moving (and fixed) parts: gears and ball bearings, wheels and axles, crankshaft and flywheel, pistons and rods. But machines are any devices that use mechanical advantage to apply force to overcome resistance (at least, historically, before the advent of devices without moving parts, such as computers). Machines assist us in performing tasks—even when they don't create energy but only transfer it, as is the case with simple machines.

The six simple machines are the lever, pulley, wheel and axle, inclined plane, wedge, and screw. Of these, the lever alone was made in humankind's image. For it may be said that the human body is a system of levers. Each human lever consists of a rigid bar (bone). Force (muscle contraction) is applied at one end of the bar to turn it about a support, or fulcrum (joint axis), in order to lift the load located at the other end of the bar. We who invented the lever are ourselves a hodgepodge of seesaws, crowbars, balance scales, nutcrackers, wheelbarrows, screen doors (operated by a short spring), catapults, and other levers.

The nuts and bolts of the body's mechanics of movement (muscle contraction producing force to move a bone around a joint's axis of rotation) can be observed in the workings of the ankle joint.

The ankle joint is the articulation of three bones: the talus (a "short bone" in the foot) and the distal tibia and the distal fibula ("long bones" in the lower leg). The ankle joint is a type of freely movable joint called a hinge joint (ginglymus); like the elbow and knee joints, it permits a wide range of movement in one plane, the anteroposterior plane, allowing the foot to move front and back. (The foot also turns inward and outward, but these aren't true ankle joint motions.)

The ankle joint allows approximately 50 degrees of extension (called, paradoxically, plantar flexion)—technically, lowering the talus bone but perhaps best explained as lowering the sole toward the ground, thereby raising the heel. And it allows approximately 15 to 20 degrees of flexion (called dorsiflexion)—technically, raising the talus bone but perhaps best explained as raising the sole so that the top of the foot moves toward the shin.

The two main extensor muscles—the gastrocnemius and the soleus—are strengthened by raising the heel and putting weight on the balls of the feet. The three flexor muscles—the tibialis anterior, extensor digitorum longus, and extensor hallucis longus—can be strengthened by walking on the heels. However, heel-raising and heel-lowering strengthening exercises can be more efficiently performed using gym equipment.

Through practicing strengthening exercises for the ankle joint and other joints, we weight-resistance yogins come to have not a theoretical but an experiential knowledge of the design, construction, operation, and care of the lever system responsible for human movement.

Just as stationary hatha yogins (seated in a meditative posture) aspire to nothing so much as becoming a living statue, weight-resistance hatha yogins aspire to become a living machine. In these goals, both hatha yogins seek to imitate Isvara, who is pure spirit, unbound by time. Unlike the Western god who created the world, intervenes in humankind's history, and answers prayers, Isvara is an archetype, a model of a yogin.

For seated yogins, the mode of being belonging to Isvara is immobility. For weight-resistance yogins, the mode of being belonging to Isvara is motion. Just as seated yogins seek to remain continuously at rest, resisting action or change, weight-resistance yogins, while securing their movements in stillness, seek to remain in motion, moving at the same speed in the same trajectory, opposing any change—whether acceleration, deceleration, altered direction, or stopping. We seek, in effect, to become a perpetual motion machine. And, indeed, some days we feel as if our movements could go on forever. Yet, like the stationary yogin, we know full well that our aspirations are ultimately futile.

As muscles continually contract against high resistance during a set, their energy source gradually becomes depleted. Some degree of discomfort (and maybe even anxiety) arises. Ultimately, the muscles become no longer capable of concentrically contracting. We've reached muscle failure, the point where we can't go on any more, where we can no longer move the resistance. The set must be terminated. (Temporary exhaustion is, of course, our fitness goal. Besides, after resting for a couple of minutes, the energy source begins to be replaced. And after a two-day rest, it's fully restored.)

Nevertheless, during the set we experience a trace of motion untouched by defilement—enough for us to have a glimmer of our true self, which is the pure spirit of Isvara. By practicing with utmost attention and precision, we make our weight-resistance yoga into *isvarapranidhana*—a contemplation of, an act of surrender to, an inhabiting of Isvara, the Divine Spirit. By these means, the practice of a coarse physical discipline—weight lifting, of all things!—becomes an acceptance of the presence of the divine in all of our actions.

On Pleasurable Repetition

Standing Heel Raise, Seated Heel Raise, and Weighted Toe Raise

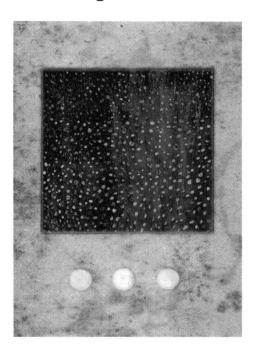

The mindless repetition of mantras, especially by the uninitiated can hardly lead to enlightenment or bliss. We must be intensely attentive in order to . . . realize the ultimate Being-Consciousness-Bliss.

—GEORG FEUERSTEIN, *THE YOGA TRADITION*

The two major calf muscles—the gastrocnemius (the prominent, two-headed muscle that shapes the back of the lower leg) and the soleus (the muscle directly underneath and slightly wider than the gastrocnemius)—come together in the Achilles tendon, which attaches to the heel bone. They provide the final push in propelling the body forward and upward. Conditioned shin muscles (at the front of the lower leg) prevent shin splints and calf injuries (by balancing the development of the calf muscles).

The calf muscles are strengthened by performing the heel raise—raising the heel of the foot (or lowering the sole of the foot) in ankle joint extension. The effect on the gastrocnemius is greatest in the standing heel raise, when the knee is straight; more work is placed on the soleus in the seated heel raise, when the knee is bent. The shin muscles are strengthened by performing the toe raise—raising the front of the foot toward the shin in ankle joint flexion. What could be simpler than these three exercises, which demand only the slightest of movements?

Yet, as I can testify from my practice, it takes a while to get the movements of these exercises right. The rear of the foot in the heel raise and the front of the foot in the toe raise need to be slowly raised and lowered in a wide range of motion. For some reason, performing these simple movements slowly and accurately doesn't come easily; we tend to rush and limit the movement. Eventually, though, we master the exercises. The struggle of getting the movement just so is over. The activity becomes always the same.

Which is exactly what many people find deadly about weight lifting. It's repetitive. Composed of a bunch of exercises performed the same way day after day, it lacks the challenge of having to adapt to changing situations found in most sports, from basketball's fast break to golf's varied terrain. No wonder many people find weight lifting boring.

But dreariness isn't inherent to weight lifting or to any other repetitive activity; what makes repetition disagreeable is our grown-up attitude toward it. For, as young children know and adults forget, "repetition, the re-experiencing of something identical," as Sigmund Freud understood, "is clearly in itself a source of pleasure."[1] Freud contrasted this pleasurable repetition, which provides comfort and satisfaction in the familiar, to both the restless quest for new experiences and the unconscious compulsion to repeat the events of childhood, which, with its "hint of possession by some 'daemonic' power," disregards the pleasure principle in every way.[2] The example that he gives of a pleasurably repeated experience is listening over and over again to the same story told exactly the same way:

> Indeed, it is hardly possible to persuade an adult who has very much enjoyed reading a book to re-read it immediately. Novelty is always the condition of enjoyment. . . . [But] if a child has been told a nice story, he will insist on hearing it over and over again rather than a new one; and he will remorselessly stipulate that the repetition shall be an identical one.[3]

During weight-resistance yoga practice, you might say that the body itself is retelling or reenacting the same story by repeating the same movements: the story of making old things new.

Just as when our eyes become accustomed to the darkness in a room, we see the room fill up with objects, when we set ourselves to doing a weight-resistance exercise exactly so, we find that we notice all the rich details demanded by the exercise. Accordingly, we move designated bony parts precisely and rhythmically (placing the movements and respiration in accord) and keep the rest of the body still. For most of us, this unnatural attentiveness to an exercise—this dwelling in the moving-yet-still body—slows down time. We find ourselves in the present, calmly observing our activity. And then, most astonishingly: the exercise becomes new, as if we were doing it for the first time. We're transported, like a traveler who arrives for the first time in a foreign city, transfixed by the trifles of everyday life there.

When we experience this kind of pleasurable repetition, in psychoanalytic terms we're reconciling Thanatos, the death instinct, with Eros, the life instinct. (The death instinct is defined by Freud as the primal will not only to repeat activities but also to attain tension-free inactivity and to affirm death.) "[If] man could enjoy the life proper to his species," writes classics scholar Norman O. Brown, building on Freud's insights, "the regressive fixation to the past would dissolve; the restless quest for novelty would be reabsorbed into the desire for pleasurable repetition; the desire to Become would be reabsorbed into the desire to Be."[4]

In yogic philosophical terms, the two opposites, death and life, are transcended in death-in-life. As yoga scholar Mircea Eliade observes: "The yogin attains deliverance; like a dead man, he has no more relation with life; he is 'dead in life.' He is the *jivan-mukti,* the 'liberated in life.' He no longer lives in time and under the domination of time, but in an eternal present."[5]

Released from the unsatisfactory cycle of compulsively seeking pleasure, the weight-resistance *jivan-mukti* replaces escapades with ritual repetition. Just as in sexual union and some forms of prayer, the regulation and repetition of bodily motions and breathing in weight-resistance yoga practice become an embodied chanting of the name of the divine, clearing the self of all else except the divine.

MEDITATION
ON SAVASANA

■ **On Contentment—Savasana**

Savasana only brings about great relief when it's preceded by the great effort of conditioning exercises—in the case of weight-resistance yoga, arduous strengthening exercises. If we hadn't just been near our physical limits, there would be no release now. For this reason, be grateful for the preceding difficulties of your exertion—so grateful, in fact, that you can let go of any disappointments over your performance.

On Contentment
Savasana

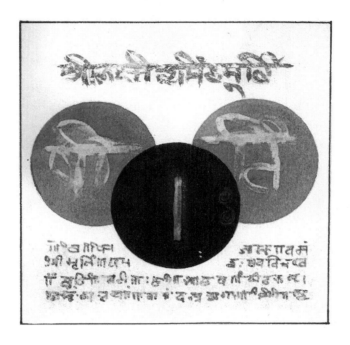

*To the poet, to the philosopher, to the saint, all things are friendly
and sacred, all events profitable, all days holy, all men divine.*

—Ralph Waldo Emerson, "History"

Lie on your back on the floor in Savasana, Corpse Pose, with your arms at your sides and your hands palms down.

Contract your pelvic floor (the area between your rectum and genitals) and release it. Contract your genital region, as if you were delaying an urgent need to urinate, and then relax the area. Tighten your abdominal region and flatten the small of your back. Relax your stomach. Slightly arch your lower back and squeeze your buttocks, while stretching from your groin to your chest. Let your back down and relax your buttocks. Your lumbar spine should once again have its neutral curve.

Slightly bend your knees, while pressing your feet flat to the floor. Tighten your back thighs. Relax your back thighs. Press your legs into the floor and tighten your front thighs and kneecaps. Relax them.

Point your feet down. Make your toes gnarled. Tighten your calves. Relax your feet and calves. Point your feet up and stiffen your toes. Tighten your shins. Relax your feet and shins. Let your feet and legs slightly drop away from each other.

Roll your shoulders forward and tighten your chest. Release your shoulders and relax your chest. Pull your shoulders back, press your upper arms into the floor, and squeeze your shoulder blades together. Release your shoulders and relax your upper back. Scrunch up your shoulders. Release your shoulders. Tighten your forearms and, with your hands still facing palm down, make a tight fist. Slowly rotate your arms outward, gradually relaxing your arms and hands. Your hands should be open with your palms facing up.

Make monkey faces. Then, while keeping your mouth closed, relax your jaw. Let your eyes sink into their sockets. Soften your brow.

Notice your breathing. The actions of the respiratory muscles are life sustaining. Like cardiac muscle and smooth muscle of the digestive tract (after we ingest food), respiratory muscle contracts involuntarily and continuously, while we're awake or asleep, throughout our life. Yet, like other skeletal muscle, respiratory muscle can be contracted voluntarily and episodically: unlike the beating of the heart, or peristalsis, breathing can be consciously stopped—for a short time. This characteristic (the quality of being *somewhat* controlled) places breathing between the voluntary and involuntary activities of the body—between, you might say, will and fate. That is to say: breathing is like the journey of life.

Savasana only brings about great relief when it's preceded by the great effort of conditioning exercises—in the case of weight-resistance yoga, arduous strengthening exercises. If we hadn't just been near our physical limits, there would be no release now. For this reason, be grateful for the preceding difficulties of your exertion—so grateful, in fact, that you can let go of any disappointments over your performance. *I could've lifted more. I rushed to get it over with. I was distracted and disengaged.* Don't regret anything about the exercising. For if you can accept what transpired while exercising, then, by extension, you can accept what's transpired in your life.

Accept the ups and downs of your entire life for where they've taken you. Don't regret the past. Don't have fantasies of great change in the future. Accept your life for what you've brought to it and what's been given to you by forces out of your hands. Your life's journey, like the very breath you're taking, is a mix of will and fate.

The notion that we should be satisfied with our life is often dismissed. But how rarely are we truly satisfied with our life! Where does wishing things were different get us, anyway, other than make us feel some degree of despair? When we're happy, don't we feel we have no wishes for things to be other than what they are at that moment? This is what's meant by *samtosha*, contentment, one of the five observances required of all aspirants to yoga.

Not that we shouldn't have desires. To find shade on a hot sunny day. To be fit and healthy. To establish a career. To find a suitable companion. To provide for our family. To wish others well. To serve others. All these desires should be met. They're what a full life is about. They're all accomplished by making necessary subtle and small, as well as mighty and difficult, adjustments to the everyday world.

But during the weight-resistance yoga session, especially during Savasana, we withdraw from the everyday world. During this time, at the deepest level of our existence, we don't wish anything were different. We don't wish we were different. We don't wish the life we lead were different. We're content with our lot in life.

Slightly stir. Gently wiggle your toes and fingers. Slightly roll from side to side. Turn to your right side. Place your right forearm and left hand on the floor. Push up. Come to a sitting position with your legs crossed and face forward. Make sure you're seated on your haunches. Keep your back aligned, and press your knees to the floor (if necessary, sit on towels or blocks to elevate your trunk and lower your legs). Place your hands in anjali mudra. Close your eyes. Observe your breath for a few moments. Open your eyes. Soon you will return to the everyday world. Go and take care of the things that need to be done. *Namaste.*

NOTES

Preface:
My Journey to Weight-Resistance Yoga

1. K. V. Iyer, *Muscle Cult: A Pro-Em to My System* (Bangalore City, India: Bangalore Press, 1930), 42.
2. K. V. Iyer, *Chemical Changes in Physical Exercise* (Bangalore City, India: Bangalore Press, 1943), iii.
3. Ibid., 3.
4. David L. Chapman, *Sandow the Magnificent: Eugen Sandow and the Beginnings of Bodybuilding* (Urbana and Chicago: University of Illinois Press, 1994), 160.
5. Yehudi Menuhin, foreword to *Light on Yoga,* by B. K. S. Iyengar, rev. ed. (New York: Schocken Books, 1979), 12.
6. B. K. S. Iyengar, *The Tree of Yoga* (1988; repr., Boston: Shambhala, 2002), 46.
7. Karl Baier, "On the philosophical dimensions of âsana," *BKS Iyengar Yoga Teachers' Association News Magazine* (Winter 1994): 18.
8. Svatmarama, *Hatha Yoga Pradipika,* trans. Pancham Sinh (Delhi: Sri Satguru Publications, 1981), 57. (Originally published in 1915.)

Introduction:
The Path of Weight-Resistance Yoga

1. Nicholas A. Ratamess, et. al., "Progression Models in Resistance Training for Healthy Adults," *Medicine & Science in Sports & Exercise* 41, no. 3 (March 2009): 688.

2. Gheranda, *Gheranda-Samhita* (New Delhi: Munshiram Manoharlal Publishers, 2001), 37. (First published in 1914–1915 by Panini Office, Allahabad.)
3. Gorakhnath, quoted in Mircea Eliade, *Yoga: Immortality and Freedom* (Princeton, N.J.: Princeton University Press, 1958), 228. The original source for this quote is George W. Briggs, trans., *Gorakhnath and the Kanphata Yogis* (Delhi: Motilal Banarsidass, 1938), 287–88.

Chapter 2. Safe and Efficient Effort

1. K. V. Iyer, *Physique & Figure* (Bangalore City, India: Bangalore Press, 1940), 85–86.

Chapter 4. Movement in Stillness

1. Steven Vogel, *Prime Mover: A Natural History of Muscle* (New York: W. W. Norton & Company, 2001), 27.

Chapter 5. Great Effort

1. Mircea Eliade, *Yoga: Immortality and Freedom* (Princeton, N.J.: Princeton University Press, 1969), 55.
2. Ibid., 58.

Chapter 14. Meditations on the Shoulder Joint

1. Mabel E. Todd, *The Thinking Body* (1937; repr.,

Princeton, N.J.: Princeton Book Company, 1968), 1.

2. Dona Holleman, ed., *Yoga Darsana of B.K.S. Iyengar, London, 1970–1974,* vol. II (self-published, 1987), 125.

3. B. K. S. Iyengar, *The Tree of Yoga* (1988; repr. Boston: Shambhala, 2002), 70.

4. Karl Baier, "Iyengar and the Yoga Tradition," *BKS Iyengar Yoga Teachers' Association News Magazine* (Winter 1995): 30.

5. Mircea Eliade, *Yoga: Immortality and Freedom* (Princeton, N.J.: Princeton University Press, 1969), 98.

6. David Gordon White, "'Open' and 'Closed' Models of the Human Body in Indian Medical and Yogic Traditions," *Asian Medicine: Tradition and Modernity* 2, no. 1, (2006): 2.

7. Eliade, *Yoga: Immortality and Freedom,* 97.

8. Ibid.

Chapter 15. Meditations on the Elbow Joint

1. David Michael Levin, *The Body's Recollection of Being: Phenomenological Psychology and the Deconstruction of Nihilism* (London: Routledge & Kegan Paul, 1985), 129.

2. Ibid.

3. Steven Vogel, *Prime Mover: A Natural History of Muscle* (New York: W. W. Norton & Company, 2001), 19.

4. Albert Szent-Györgyi, quoted in *Profiles in Science, The Albert Szent-Gyorgyi Papers,* "Szeged, 1931–1947: Vitamin C, Muscles, and WWII," Bethesda, Md.: National Library of Medicine, http://profiles.nlm.nih.gov/ps/display/Main (accessed July 12, 2011).

5. Morton Oliver, *Eating the Sun: How Plants Power the Planet* (New York: HarperCollins, 2008), xvi.

6. Alain Daniélou, *The Gods of India: Hindu Polytheism* (New York: Inner Traditions, 1985), 9. (Reissued under the title *The Myths and Gods of India* in 1991 by Inner Traditions, Rochester, Vt.)

Chapter 16. Meditations on the Shoulder Girdle

1. Charles Darwin, *The Expression of Emotion in Man and Animals* (London: Penguin Group, 2009), 248. (Originally published in 1872; this edition based on the 2nd ed. published in 1890.)

2. Ibid., 247.

3. Ibid., 248.

Chapter 17. Meditations on the Trunk (Vertebral Column and Abdominal Wall)

1. Stuart Sovatsky, *Words from the Soul: Time, East/West Spirituality, and Psychotherapeutic Narrative* (Albany: State University of New York Press, 1998), 26.

2. B. K. S. Iyengar, *The Tree of Yoga* (1988, repr., Boston: Shambhala, 2002), 50.

3. Mel C. Siff, *Fact and Fallacies of Fitness* (Denver, Colo.: self-published, 2003), 166.

4. Patanjali: *Yoga Aphorisms,* trans. and commentator Ernest E. Wood, in *Practical Yoga, Ancient and Modern* (New York: E. P. Dutton, 1948), 110.

5. Mircea Eliade, *Yoga: Immortality and Freedom* (Princeton, N.J.: Princeton University Press, 1969), 96.

Chapter 18. Meditations on the Hip Joint and Pelvic Girdle

1. Aristotle, *The Works of Aristotle,* vol. 5., *De Partibus Animalium* [On the Parts of Animals], book 4, eds. J. A. Smith and W. D. Ross, trans. William Ogle (London: Oxford University Press, 1949),

689b, 1–27. (Quotation abridged and edited by the author.)

2. Irwin W. Straus, *Phenomenological Psychology* (New York: Basic Books, 1966), 143.

3. Mabel E. Todd, *The Thinking Body* (1937; repr., Princeton, N.J.: Princeton Book Company, 1968), 1.

4. Straus, *Phenomenological Psychology,* 148.

Chapter 19. Meditations on the Knee Joint

1. René Descartes, *Treatise of Man,* trans. T. S. Hall (Cambridge, Mass.: Harvard University Press, 1972), 34. (Originally published in French in 1664.)

2. Jean Couch with Nell Weaver, *Runner's World Yoga Book* (Mountain View, Calif.: Runner's World Books, 1979), 167.

3. Karlfried Graf Von Dürckheim, *Hara: The Vital Centre of Man* (London: George Allen & Unwin, 1962), 27. (Reissued in 2004 by Inner Traditions, Rochester, Vt.)

4. Ellington Darden, *The Nautilus Bodybuilding Book* (Chicago: Contemporary Books, 1982), 75.

5. Ibid.

6. K. V. Iyer, *Physique & Figure* (Bangalore City, India: Bangalore Press, 1940), 81.

7. Ibid., 85–86.

8. Vācaspatimiśra, quoted in Mircea Eliade, *Yoga: Immortality and Freedom* (Princeton, N.J.: Princeton University Press, 1969), 51.

Chapter 20. Meditations on the Ankle Joint

1. Sigmund Freud, *Beyond the Pleasure Principle,* trans. James Strachey (New York: Bantam Books, 1959), 66.

2. Ibid., 67.

3. Ibid., 66.

4. Norman O. Brown, *Life Against Death: The Psychoanalytical Meaning of History* (New York: Vintage Books, 1959), 93.

5. Mircea Eliade, *Yoga: Immortality and Freedom* (Princeton, N.J.: Princeton University Press, 1969), 93–94.

INDEX

Page numbers in *italics* refer to illustrations.